T0259252

Endoscopy

Guest Editor

MARYANN G. RADLINSKY, DVM, MS

VETERINARY CLINICS OF NORTH AMERICA: SMALL ANIMAL PRACTICE

www.vetsmall.theclinics.com

September 2009 • Volume 39 • Number 5

SAUNDERS an imprint of ELSEVIER, Inc.

W.B. SAUNDERS COMPANY
A Division of Elsevier Inc.

1600 John F. Kennedy Blvd. • Suite 1800 • Philadelphia, PA 19103-2899

http://www.vetsmall.theclinics.com

VETERINARY CLINICS OF NORTH AMERICA: SMALL ANIMAL PRACTICE Volume 39, Number 5
September 2009 ISSN 0195-5616, ISBN-13: 978-1-4377-1286-5, ISBN-10: 1-4377-1286-X

Editor: John Vassallo; j.vassallo@elsevier.com
Developmental Editor: Donald Mumford

Veterinary Clinics of North America: Small Animal Practice (ISSN 0195-5616) is published bimonthly (For Post Office use only: volume 39 issue 5 of 6) by Elsevier Inc., 360 Park Avenue South, New York, NY 10010-1710. Months of issue are January, March, May, July, September, and November. Application to mail at periodicals postage rates is pending at New York, NY and at additional mailing offices. Subscription prices are $229.00 per year (domestic individuals), $366.00 per year (domestic institutions), $114.00 per year (domestic students/residents), $303.00 per year (Canadian individuals), $450.00 per year (Canadian institutions), $336.00 per year (international individuals), $450.00 per year (international institutions), and $165.00 per year (international and Canadian students/residents). To receive student/resident rate, orders must be accompanied by name of affiliated institution, date of term, and the *signature* of program/residency coordinator on institution letterhead. Orders will be billed at individual rate until proof of status is received. Foreign air speed delivery is included in all *Clinics* subscription prices. All prices are subject to change without notice. **POSTMASTER:** Send address changes to *Veterinary Clinics of North America: Small Animal Practice*, Elsevier Health Sciences Division, Subscription Customer Service, 3251 Riverport Lane, Maryland Heights, MO 63043. Customer Service (orders, claims, online, change of address): Elsevier Periodicals Customer Service, Elsevier Health Sciences Division Subscription Customer Service 3251 Riverport Lane Maryland Heights, MO 63043. Tel: 1-800-654-2452 (U.S. and Canada); 314-447-8871 (outside U.S. and Canada). Fax: 314-447-8029. E-mail: journalscustomerservice-usa@elsevier.com (for print support); journalsonlinesupport-usa@elsevier.com (for online support).

Reprints. For copies of 100 or more of articles in this publication, please contact the Commercial Reprints Department, Elsevier Inc., 360 Park Avenue South, New York, NY 10010-1710. Tel.: 212-633-3812; Fax: 212-462-1935; E-mail: reprints@elsevier.com.

Veterinary Clinics of North America: Small Animal Practice is also published in Japanese by Inter Zoo Publishing Co., Ltd., Aoyama Crystal-Bldg 5F, 3-5-12 Kitaaoyama, Minato-ku, Tokyo 107-0061, Japan.

Veterinary Clinics of North America: Small Animal Practice is covered in *Current Contents/Agriculture, Biology and Environmental Sciences, Science Citation Index, ASCA, MEDLINE/PubMed (Index Medicus), Excerpta Medica,* and *BIOSIS.*

Printed and bound in the United Kingdom

Transferred to Digital Print 2011

Contributors

GUEST EDITOR

MARYANN G. RADLINSKY, DVM, MS
Diplomate, American College of Veterinary Surgeons; Associate Professor, Department of Small Animal Medicine and Surgery, College of Veterinary Medicine, University of Georgia, Athens, Georgia

AUTHORS

NICOLE J. BUOTE, DVM
Surgical Resident, Department of Surgery, The Animal Medical Center, New York, New York

KATE E. CREEVY, DVM, MS
Diplomate, American College of Veterinary Internal Medicine; Assistant Professor, Department of Small Animal Medicine and Surgery, College of Veterinary Medicine, University of Georgia, Athens, Georgia

LYNETTA J. FREEMAN, DVM, MS
Diplomate, American College of Veterinary Surgeons; Associate Professor of Small Animal Surgery & Biomedical Engineering, Department of Veterinary Clinical Sciences, Purdue University School of Veterinary Medicine, West Lafayette, Indiana

PHILIPP D. MAYHEW, BVM&S, MRCVS
Diplomate, American College of Veterinary Surgeons; Columbia River Veterinary Specialists, Vancouver, Washington

JANET KOVAK McCLARAN, DVM
Diplomate, American College of Veterinary Surgeons; Staff Surgeon, Department of Surgery, The Animal Medical Center, New York, New York

ERIC MONNET, DVM, PhD, FAHA
Diplomate, American College of Veterinary Surgeons and European College of Veterinary Surgeons; Professor of Small Animal Surgery, Department of Clinical Sciences, Colorado State University, Fort Collins, Colorado

MARYANN G. RADLINSKY, DVM, MS
Diplomate, American College of Veterinary Surgeons; Associate Professor, Department of Small Animal Medicine and Surgery, College of Veterinary Medicine, University of Georgia, Athens, Georgia

CLARENCE A. RAWLINGS, DVM, PhD
Diplomate, American College of Veterinary Surgeons; Professor Emeritus, Department of Small Animal Medicine and Surgery, College of Veterinary Medicine, University of Georgia, Athens, Georgia

CHAD SCHMIEDT, DVM
Diplomate, American College of Veterinary Surgeons; Assistant Professor of Small Animal Surgery, Department of Small Animal Medicine and Surgery, College of Veterinary Medicine, University of Georgia, Athens, Georgia

STEFFEN SUM, DVM
Medical Instructor, Department of Small Animal Medicine and Surgery, University of Georgia, College of Veterinary Medicine, Athens, Georgia

ANNE P. VAN LUE, DVM, PhD
Preclinical Consultant, Santa Clara, California

STEPHEN J. VAN LUE, DVM
Diplomate, American College of Veterinary Surgeons; Diplomate, European College of Veterinary Surgeons; General Manager CA, Senior Director, Surgical Research and Innovation, LyChron, LLC, Mountain View, California

CYNTHIA R. WARD, VMD, PhD
Diplomate, American College of Veterinary Internal Medicine; Associate Professor, Department of Small Animal Medicine and Surgery, College of Veterinary Medicine, University of Georgia, Athens, Georgia

ANN B. WEIL, MS, DVM
Diplomate, America College of Veterinary Anesthesiologists; Clinical Associate Professor of Anesthesiology, Department of Veterinary Clinical Sciences, School of Veterinary Medicine Purdue University, West Lafayette, Indiana

Contents

varying levels of experience have been developed to access and evaluate each anatomic region. Familiarity with appropriate indications for each procedure and normal appearance, cytology, and culture results from each region will enhance diagnostic success.

Flexible endoscopy is a valuable tool for the diagnosis of many small animal digestive tract diseases. This article provides a basic introduction to small animal gastrointestinal endoscopy including its diagnostic advantages as well as its limitations and complications. Although proficiency in endoscopic techniques can only be obtained through many hours of practice, this article should also encourage and stimulate the novice endoscopist.

Since 1999, when the author first described the research and potential applications of minimally invasive gastrointestinal surgery in animals, veterinarians have begun to apply some of these techniques in treating client owned animals. Minimally invasive surgery is advocated with diagnostic, prophylactic, and therapeutic intent. There has been a transition from a minimally invasive caseload toward the expansion of diagnostic procedures, adoption of prophylactic procedures (such as lap-assisted gastropexy), and performing more difficult therapeutic procedures. Small animal patients benefit from reduced tissue trauma and experience a rapid recovery. In this article, current research and minimally invasive gastrointestinal procedures in animals are discussed.

This article discusses several advanced laparoscopic procedures that have now been described in clinical veterinary patients. Laparoscopic-assisted cholecystostomy tube placement, laparoscopic cholecystectomy, and adrenalectomy can all be performed safely and efficiently. Case selection guidelines as well as indications, techniques, and possible complications are discussed in detail.

Laparoscopic procedures provide the advantage of decreased patient morbidity with improved visualization and rapid patient recovery. Complications associated with laparoscopic procedures are discussed. Conversion to open laparotomy may depend on a variety of factors related to the patient, procedure, and surgeon. There are few contraindications for performing laparoscopic procedures, but complications or conversions to an open laparotomy may be expected in a percentage of patients.

THE CLINICS ARE NOW AVAILABLE ONLINE!

Access your subscription at:
www.theclinics.com

Preface

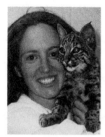

MaryAnn G. Radlinsky, DVM, MS
Guest Editor

Pet owners are increasingly aware of the advances in the practice of medicine and have come to expect the same for their pets. Endoscopy entered the veterinary field as a diagnostic tool, but the limitations of its use have been shattered in the past few years. Veterinary endoscopy started with viewing through natural orifices. There is not one that has not been "scoped;" however, entry into body cavities and other sites rapidly followed. Many interventional techniques are now well described; some have become the standard of care for certain conditions, and some are still "works in progress." The future of endoscopy is bright, to say the least. The minimal invasiveness of the techniques described in this issue has allowed veterinary patients to benefit from the rapid recovery and shortened duration of hospitalization. The development of these techniques was pioneered by physicians, and the equipment is becoming more available and specialized for veterinary use in the very large to the tiniest of patients.

This issue provides a general overview of the possibilities of endoscopy in clinical practice and will open doors for future endoscopists to develop their enthusiasm for the technique. The learning curve may be high, but many training centers exist and can jump start one to the path of minimally invasive diagnosis and therapy! Attending a continuing education experience should include hands-on practice. Further practice and application of the concepts will hone the skills required for successful endoscopy. Beginning with diagnostic techniques and slowly expanding to therapeutic ones provides a solid base upon which to grow. Starting a minimally invasive procedure and setting a time limit allows for repeated exposure to the methods used. If much progress has been made within that time limit, the procedure may be completed endoscopically; if not, convert to an open approach. Learn from every procedure—what

Vet Clin Small Anim 39 (2009) ix–x
doi:10.1016/j.cvsm.2009.06.001
0195-5616/09/$ – see front matter © 2009 Elsevier Inc. All rights reserved.

vetsmall.theclinics.com

worked well, how the technique can be improved, and if changing the approach would be beneficial—and welcome to the ever-expanding world of endoscopy!

MaryAnn G. Radlinsky, DVM, MS
Department of Small Animal Medicine and Surgery
College of Veterinary Medicine
University of Georgia
501 DW Brooks Drive
Athens, GA 30602, USA

E-mail address:
radlinsk@uga.edu (M.G. Radlinsky)

Equipment and Instrumentation in Veterinary Endoscopy

Stephen J. Van Lue, DVM[a],*, Anne P. Van Lue, DVM, PhD[b]

KEYWORDS

- Trocars • Instruments • Rigid endoscopy • Flexible endoscopy
- Laparoscopy

An endoscopic procedure uses a lighted viewing instrument (endoscope) to look inside a body cavity or organ to diagnose or treat disorders.[1] Endoscopes can be either flexible or rigid, or a hybrid combination. Rigid endoscopes are most often referred to as telescopes, and are named according to the anatomic region in which they are most used. Rigid endoscopy includes laparoscopy, thoracoscopy, rhinoscopy, cystoscopy, otoscopy, hysteroscopy, and arthroscopy. Flexible endoscopy includes bronchoscopy, endoscopy of the upper and lower gastrointestinal (GI) tracts, male urinary tract, and ureteroscopy. Endoscopic methods are also used subcutaneously in the harvest of vascular grafts for coronary artery bypass grafting procedures in humans.

The principle involves the passage of light from a source through an endoscope/telescope to illuminate a target region and display the image on a monitor by means of a camera and camera control unit. Some advanced endoscopes have the image sensor located at the endoscope's distal tip, rather than using a camera coupled to the eyepiece of the telescope, for capture and transmission of the image. These are often referred to as "chip on a stick" endoscopes, and are discussed further in a subsequent section.

Endoscopic procedures are minimally invasive in nature, and, whether using natural orifices or obtaining access through small incisions and trocars, have been found to decrease the postoperative stress response and postoperative pain compared with similar procedures performed by an open approach.[2–5] This, together with clients' desire to have their pet undergo as gentle a procedure as possible, forms the rationale behind the increasing use of endoscopy in small animal practice. There is a tremendous ongoing effort to make minimally invasive surgery less invasive through research and the development of new and improved medical devices, making the term

[a] Surgical Research and Innovation, LyChron, LLC, 2569 Wyandotte Street, Mountain View, CA 94043, USA
[b] 1150 Doyle Circle, Santa Clara, CA 95054, USA
* Corresponding author.
E-mail address: svanlue@lychron.com (S.J. Van Lue).

Vet Clin Small Anim 39 (2009) 817–837
doi:10.1016/j.cvsm.2009.06.002
0195-5616/09/$ – see front matter © 2009 Elsevier Inc. All rights reserved.

"minimally invasive" even less oxymoronic. Some examples are the advent of single-port techniques, hybrid laparoscopic procedures, and natural orifice translumenal endoscopic surgery (NOTES), with the latter's ultimate goal being incisionless surgery. NOTES, as well as other new developments, are reviewed in a subsequent article. These new devices and techniques will find their way into veterinary surgery. This article provides a general overview of the necessary equipment and instrumentation that will assist practitioners in making decisions for the incorporation of endoscopy/endoscopic surgery into their practice.

OPERATING ROOM REQUIREMENTS/SPACE

A review of aseptic principles for operating room (OR) layout is beyond the scope of this section. However, there are a few things to consider with regard to minimally invasive procedures for OR layout/design and equipment, depending on the goals and needs of the practitioner. Generally speaking, a laparoscopic or thoracoscopic procedure should only be performed in a location in which the identical procedure could be performed conventionally, with proper aseptic technique, in the event it is necessary to convert to an open approach for any reason.

When performing minimally invasive procedures (particularly laparoscopy and thoracoscopy), more space is required to accommodate the endoscopic tower, which may need to be moved or even swung in an arc a distance from the surgical table. Space for multiple monitors may also need to be considered. If a monitor is present at each end of the surgical table, adjustment in the location of anesthesia equipment may be required. Having power sockets suspended from the ceiling helps to avoid clutter and tripping hazards during the low-light periods when the equipment is in use. Additional space may be required for a larger Mayo stand which can accommodate the increased length of laparoscopic instruments as well as the conventional instruments necessary for a given procedure.

The Surgical Table

For minimally invasive procedures, exposure of the target area is critical for success, and the use of gravitational forces is the most effective means of achieving this. Although the use of gravity is often augmented by other specialized retraction instrumentation or techniques, the surgical table is the primary device that enables the operator to most efficiently employ gravitational forces. The ideal table allows the surgeon to tilt the patient laterally in either direction as well as varying degrees of head-up (known as reverse Trendelenberg position) or head-down (Trendelenberg position) positions. A key principle regarding the use of the table is to tilt the table/patient away from the desired target one wishes to visualize, particularly in a laparoscopic procedure, which encourages mobile viscera to move in a dependent fashion away from the target area(s). Thus one can appreciate the use of such a table in a laparoscopic exploratory procedure, in which all abdominal quadrants need to be examined. Generally speaking, table height will be lower during a laparoscopic procedure than a conventional procedure due to the long length of the instruments. The table must accommodate the desired height to avoid shoulder pain or other repetitive strain injuries which can result from protracted elevation of the hands while performing laparoscopic surgery.

Trendelenberg tables can be expensive, and, for procedures in which the precise position of the patient is known for effective visualization of the target, a standard table can be tilted before the procedure. Along with patient positioning devices, the patient can be secured to reduce the risk of falling. Undue pressure on the limbs from security straps should be avoided; padded straps are available commercially. As one begins to perform more advanced procedures, a Trendelenberg table is essential.

TOWER
Cart

With the exception of some portable endoscopy units, all of the components referred to as the tower are arranged on a mobile cart (**Fig. 1**). The cart should enable the various components to be readily accessed by OR personnel, and key analog or digital data displays should be easily visualized by the anesthesiologist and surgeons if not displayed on the video monitor. The cart should be of sturdy construction of a hospital grade material that can withstand regular cleaning and disinfection. In addition, the wheels should be lockable, and the cart should not be top heavy when fully loaded. Many carts have locking doors and drawers. Having a cart that provides electrical plug-ins for the various components is also helpful, and having the entire tower operate from a single on/off master switch, and plugging into a single socket, helps to avoid clutter and enables easier movement of the tower during a procedure. Typically, the video display is located at the top of the cart, or may be on a mechanical arm, which affords the operators more versatility in monitor position. The cart should also securely accommodate a CO_2 tank as a primary source of insufflation gas, or as a backup in the event a central gas supply malfunctions.

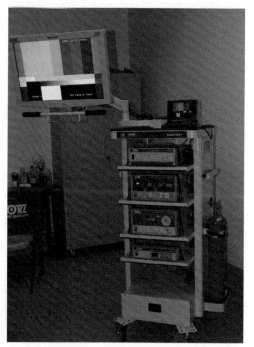

Fig. 1. Rigid endoscopy tower including (from top to bottom) a 31′ LCD HD monitor, supplemental HD portable digital video recorder, digital recording unit for still photos and video segments, insufflator, xenon light source, and camera control unit.

Telescope

The telescope uses glass lenses to direct light by way of a fiberoptic bundle to illuminate the target area and the eyepiece. In conventional telescopes, a series of lenses are embedded in an air medium, whereas in the Hopkins rod lens telescopes, the lenses have been replaced with glass rods separated by small negative air lenses (**Fig. 2**). This system allows more light to be transmitted to the tip of the telescope; it yields greater magnification and provides greater depth and a wider field of view than the conventional system. Most telescopes sold today use Hopkins technology. Magnification (zoom) can be achieved optically with lenses, digitally through the camera control unit, or by moving the telescope closer to the target structure. Digital zoom amplifies the existing pixels in the image; no loss of light occurs, but there is an overall loss of contrast. Optical zoom preserves contrast, but, just as with a high-power astronomical telescope, there is a net loss of light. Given the close quarters of working within a body cavity with a xenon light source, this is not normally a significant factor.

Typically, the telescope is used in conjunction with a camera that captures and transmits the image to a video monitor, but many basic procedures can still be performed with the use of the eyepiece alone. The disadvantage of not using a video camera is that the operator is not ergonomically situated in a manner conducive to using both hands to operate instruments. Thus, a cameraless technique is limited to basic diagnostic procedures and elementary biopsy techniques. Further, without the use of a video camera, others are not able to view the procedure in real time, nor are they able to function as surgical assistants, and a video record of the procedure cannot be created for review and documentation or educational purposes.

The most important considerations in choosing a telescope are diameter, angle of view, and length. The greater the diameter of the telescope, the greater amount of light that can be conducted for illumination, and the larger the field of view. Thus a larger diameter endoscope may be more useful during a case involving a larger animal, in which panoramic views across the peritoneal cavity may be desired. Telescopes are made in several different diameters ranging from 1.2 mm to 10 mm. A 5-mm telescope is sufficient for most small animal patients for laparoscopy and thoracoscopy, whereas for most other purposes (ie, arthroscopy, cystoscopy, rhinoscopy) a 2.7-mm telescope (or smaller) is preferable. For the smaller telescopes, a protective sheath is recommended to avoid damage to the sensitive structures within the telescope.

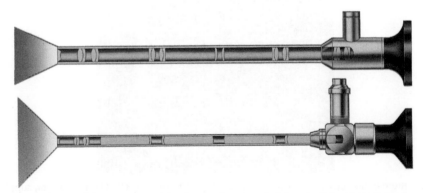

Fig. 2. Hopkins rod lens system with glass rods separated by small "negative" air lenses. (*Courtesy of* Karl Storz GmbH & Co. KG, Tuttlingen, Germany.)

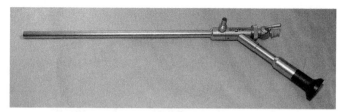

Fig. 3. Operating endoscope with instrument channel.

A rigid telescope with a working channel for the passage of an instrument is known as an operating endoscope, and is adequate for diagnostic viewing or simple biopsy procedures (**Fig. 3**).

Telescopes have various viewing angles typically ranging from 0° to 45°, but may range up to 90° or even 120° (**Fig. 4**). A wider viewing angle enables the operator to see over anatomic structures and around corners where the view would otherwise be obstructed with a 0° telescope, and helps to prevent the telescope from interfering with other operative instruments.[6] By rotating an angled telescope along its axis (by rotating the light guide cable), a larger field of view is obtained, enabling the operator to look up, down, left, and right with the telescope in the same axial position. Recently, a telescope was introduced that eliminates the need for the surgeon to choose a particular viewing angle at the outset of a procedure, or the need to change endoscopes during a procedure if a change in viewing angle is required. This telescope, called the Cameleon (Karl Storz GmbH & Co. KG, Tuttlingen, Germany), provides for adjustment of the viewing angle by turning a dial located at the proximal end of the telescope (**Fig. 5**). The 0° scope is the simplest to use, because one sees precisely what is aimed at, but, with a little practice, an angled telescope is much more useful, particularly for major procedures in the abdomen and thorax, as well as arthroscopy, in which mobility is limited by the bony structures surrounding the telescope. A 30°,

Viewing Angle

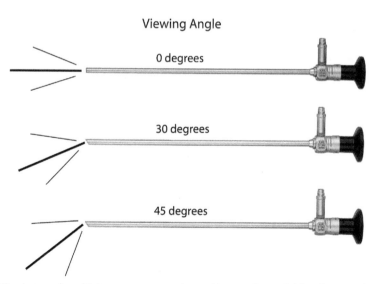

Fig. 4. Viewing angles of telescopes commonly used in veterinary rigid endoscopy. (*Courtesy of* Karl Storz GmbH & Co. KG, Tuttlingen, Germany.)

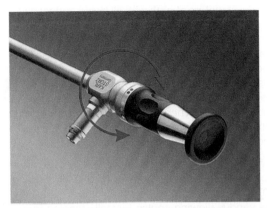

Fig. 5. The Cameleon Telescope (Karl Storz GmbH & Co. KG, Tuttlingen, Germany) provides for adjustment of the viewing angle by turning a dial located at the proximal end of the telescope. (*Courtesy of* Karl Storz GmbH & Co. KG, Tuttlingen, Germany.)

5-mm telescope is probably the most versatile for laparoscopic and thoracoscopic procedures in small animals.

The length of the telescope is largely predetermined by the chosen diameter, and varies from 10 cm to 35 cm. One should not attempt to perform an endoscopic procedure with too short a telescope, as it may not be able to be positioned close enough to the target structures to illuminate them sufficiently, or provide sufficient magnification to operate effectively.

At the outset of the procedure, a telescope will often fog as a result of condensation produced on the lens due to the temperature difference between the OR and the internal environment of the patient. This condensation will subside as the endoscope warms, but may be mitigated before the procedure by using a commercially available, sterile surfactant solution to prevent fogging, or by using a commercially available endoscope warmer. An autoclaved stainless steel thermos filled with warm saline is also effective. During the procedure, minor fogging or fouling of the lens often is addressed by gently swiping the distal tip of the scope across a tissue interface, such as omentum.

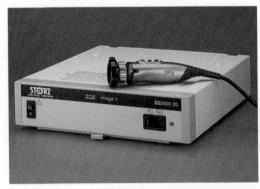

Fig. 6. Camera and camera control unit. (*Courtesy of* Karl Storz GmbH & Co. KG, Tuttlingen, Germany.)

Camera

Overall image quality significantly impacts an operator's ability to perform an endoscopic procedure, whether for diagnostic or therapeutic purposes, and a high-quality camera and camera control unit is extremely important (**Fig. 6**). A great deal of advancement has occurred and is currently ongoing in the field of high-end surgical optics. Camera selection was once limited to either a single-chip or 3-chip system, which refers directly to the number of charge-coupled devices (CCDs) in the camera system. In a 3-chip system, a beam splitter sends the red, green, and blue components of the image to each respective CCD. Three-CCD cameras generally provide better image quality than single-CCD systems because they have more lines of resolution, and are typically more expensive. However, many single-chip cameras are readily available and affordable, and are adequate for many procedures. Both of these cameras acquire the initial image data in an analog format, which is then converted to a digital signal.

Recently, high definition (HD) has become available in endoscopic cameras, with a few select systems offering full HD (1080 pixels in a 16 × 9 aspect ratio). Standard definition has a resolution of 720 × 576, whereas full HD provides 5 times the resolution at 1920 × 1080. The image obtained with these cameras, particularly those in the 16 × 9 widescreen aspect ratio, often emulates a three-dimensional image during viewing on the video monitor, which is partly due to the image mimicking the orientation/horizontal spacing of the human eye. Because of the wider field of view, the operator has the advantage of visualizing the instruments more readily when they are positioned, or are being introduced from, the extreme lateral aspects of the viewing field (**Fig. 7**). This advantage alone makes endoscopic suturing easier when using an HD system in widescreen format. As with all new technologies, these cameras are expensive, but with newer technology under development, these systems will become standard.

Light Source

The light source for endoscopic procedures typically uses halogen or xenon bulbs; the higher the wattage, the greater the intensity of light. For illuminating smaller anatomic spaces, such as in arthroscopic procedures, a lower-intensity system may be adequate. However, in larger animals, a 300 W light source is preferred for panoramic

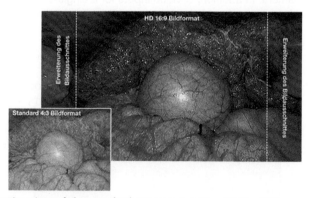

Fig. 7. Comparative view of the standard 4:3 aspect ratio with the 16:9 aspect ratio (widescreen format). Note increased lateral area of view. (*Courtesy of* Karl Storz GmbH & Co. KG, Tuttlingen, Germany.)

viewing in the chest and abdomen. In addition to the type of light source used, the diameter of the endoscope (and fiberoptic transmission capacity) also influences how much light is available. Older systems may not have an automatic iris adjustment feature, and therefore the light intensity may need to be manually adjusted accordingly, depending on the above factors as well as the pigmentary characteristics of the tissue or organ, and distance of the endoscope tip from the target site. Darker tissues and blood tend to absorb light. If a tissue being illuminated is highly reflective, the intensity of the light source may need to be reduced to prevent a whiteout.

Modern light sources track bulb life, which makes it easier for the operators to gauge when replacement should be conducted without the loss of illumination during a procedure. Nevertheless, it is recommended that a replacement bulb always be available to obviate the need to convert to an open procedure due to bulb burnout. Another approach is to have a more economical backup light source readily available, which may already be used in the practice of other diagnostic procedures, such as otoscopy.

Light Guide Cable

The light guide cable is a fiberoptic bundle that conducts light from the light source to the endoscope. A poor-quality or damaged cable will negatively influence the amount of light available for illumination during viewing. Be certain that the connectors at both ends are kept clean. Individual fiberoptic strands in the bundle may eventually break and significantly reduce light-transmission capacity. Before committing to purchase a used light-guide cable, determine the relative number of damaged fibers by connecting the cable to the light source (or holding one end of the cable up to a bright light) while simultaneously shining the light emitted from the other end onto a wall.[6] Broken individual fibers will appear as black spots, whereas more significant damage may appear as coalescing black areas (**Fig. 8**). Practice caution in placing the bare end of a fully illuminated cable, because significant heat can be generated and can create an intraoperative fire hazard or injure the patient.

Monitor

It is important to realize that a high-end monitor will not make a poor-quality image from damaged or worn equipment look better. At a minimum, the video monitor should have 500 lines of resolution if using a single-chip camera, and 750 lines of resolution if using a 3-chip camera. In addition, S-video inputs for a single-chip camera and RGB inputs for a 3-chip camera should also be present to maximize image quality. For full

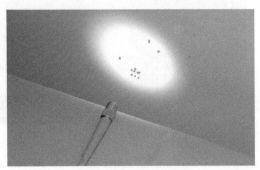

Fig. 8. Broken fibers will manifest as coalescing black areas or individual black spots when the light is shown on a wall.

HD systems, a high-resolution, flat panel, LCD monitor capable of displaying in 16:9 aspect ratio (widescreen) is required to realize the full benefits of the expanded lateral viewing capability as well as the perceived three-dimensional effect, which results from the wide aspect ratio, increased resolution, and color separation.

Insufflator

The insufflator is a computer-controlled electronic pump that displays and maintains the intra-abdominal pressure (insufflation pressure) at a preset value. The total amount of CO_2 insufflated, flow rate, and remaining tank pressure can also be monitored on most units (**Fig. 9**). Suction not only evacuates fluid, blood, or smoke, but may also cause a sudden drop in insufflation pressure, thereby obscuring the image. Because suction is often used at more critical periods of a procedure to assist with visualization, sudden loss of insufflation pressure simply compounds the problem. Hence, insufflators have become more advanced and flow-rate capabilities have increased dramatically. For advanced procedures, a high-flow insufflator, with a CO_2-flow of up to 20 L/min, is essential.

Whether using a Veress needle, or an open Hasson (or variation thereof) approach, at the outset of initiating insufflation, the pressure should be low, with a high flow rate on the insufflator display, thereby reflecting the instillation of the CO_2 gas into the large potential space of the peritoneal cavity. If pressure is initially high, all stopcocks should be checked to ensure they are in the open position. If pressure still remains high, it is possible the Veress needle or cannula is not within the desired tissue space.

Recording Capability

The recording of still images, video clips, and entire surgical procedures is now easy with the advancements that have accompanied the integration of digital media recorders into the operating room. A standard VCR/VHS format is also readily affordable and available, but, for high-volume documentation and archiving, storage space can become problematic. In addition, future review and editing are more labor intensive with older VHS recording systems.

A digital recording system (**Fig. 10**) can accommodate various output formats, enabling video clips in MPEG format or stills in JPEG, GIF, or TIFF to be stored locally on a hard-drive contained within the recording device, exported to an external drive, burned to a DVD or CD ROM, or directed to a network location. Thus the procedure(s) and various portions thereof can be readily recalled or shown in real time, being displayed in conference rooms, offices, or adjacent operating rooms during a training

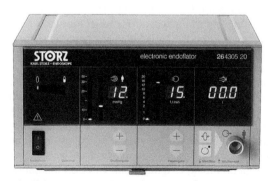

Fig. 9. Insufflator with digital display of relative CO_2 tank pressure, insufflation pressure, flow rate, and total volume. (*Courtesy of* Karl Storz GmbH & Co. KG, Tuttlingen, Germany.)

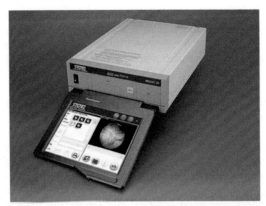

Fig. 10. Digital recording system with various output formats, enabling video clips in MPEG format or stills in JPEG, GIF, or TIFF to be stored locally on a hard drive contained within the recording device, exported to an external drive, burned to a DVD or CDROM, or directed to a network location. (*Courtesy of* Karl Storz GmbH & Co. KG, Tuttlingen, Germany.)

session, with flat-panel monitors. With simple network archiving in a practice setting, the practitioner can review aspects of the procedure in the examination room, with a client, on a wall-mounted flat-panel video monitor. These same capabilities essentially form the foundation of telesurgery, whereby individuals from around the globe can participate in or observe a surgical procedure simultaneously. A word of caution: most digital recorders enable immediate playback of a stored video clip, and, if it is displayed and reviewed on the primary viewing monitor during a surgical case, an accidental injury to the patient could occur. The surgeons must be made aware of any play back of video clips on the primary viewing monitor during a live case, so they do not view the prerecorded video on the monitor, and thereby respond to a grossly inaccurate portrayal of precisely how their instruments are engaged within the patient.

TROCARS

A trocar is the device that enables smooth passage of endoscopic instruments or an imaging device across a tissue plane or body-wall boundary. A traditional trocar typically consists of a cannula (hollow portion) and an obturator with a sharp tip, which protrudes from the cannula tip, for penetrating tissue. Other bladeless cannulas use a threaded screw mechanism or have protrusions at the distal tip that perform blunt dissection when pressure is applied with a twisting motion. Examples of different types of trocars are shown in **Fig. 11.** Many trocars also are known as optical trocars, meaning that the endoscope can be placed into the lumen of the cannula and the trocar's insertion progress can be viewed on the video monitor (**Fig. 12**).

In addition to enabling the smooth passage of instruments, most trocars, particularly for laparoscopic use, have a valve feature that seals around the instrument shaft, and also seals the cannula when no instrument is present, to preserve insufflation pressure. Loss of insufflation pressure can result in loss of visualization of the surgical target, making valves a critical feature. Generally, CO_2 insufflation is maintained by connecting the insufflation tubing to a stopcock valve on the cannula.

Trocars typically range from 3 mm to 12 mm in diameter. Much larger sizes (up to several centimeters in diameter) are available for placement of specialized

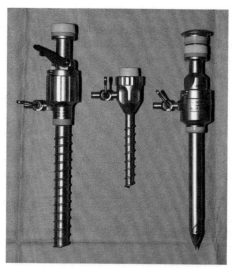

Fig.11. Reusable trocars with sharp obturator or threaded cannulas in 5 mm and 10 mm sizes.

instrumentation such as staplers or tissue morcellators, and accommodate the removal of large amounts of resected tissue (bowel loops, uterus, kidney, and so forth).

Trocars with spring-loaded safety shields that cover the sharp obturator tip following penetration of a tissue boundary have fallen somewhat out of favor, and according to the US Food and Drug Administration (FDA), may no longer be referred to as safety shields in the product description, as over time they have not been shown to be more safe in clinical use.[7] These trocars are very useful, and are readily available, but one should not assume that injury to underlying anatomic structures cannot occur. In humans, insertion of the primary trocar causes most of the reported injuries and accounts for 83% of vascular injuries, 75% of bowel injuries, and 50% of local hemorrhage injuries.[8] Most studies report an overall complication rate from the use of trocars of approximately 3%, with the most serious complications happening following vascular injury.[8–11]

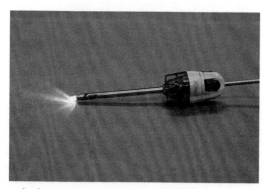

Fig.12. The light from the laparoscope can be seen shining through this optical trocar's distal viewing lens, which enables the operator to view the trocar's progress during insertion.

In contrast to laparoscopic cannulas, those used for thoracoscopic procedures are much shorter, use a blunt obturator, and may be rigid or flexible (**Fig. 13**). A rigid cannula may be preferable when a rigid telescope is passed through a cannula that is in an intercostal space. The telescope can be easily damaged when manipulated during the procedure if the adjacent ribs create a fulcrum of force on the shaft. Otherwise, a flexible cannula is sufficient and provides for less trauma to the intercostal muscles, vessels, and nerves. Thoracic cannulas do not always have a valve feature, as selective endobronchial intubation of the contralateral lung and atelectasis of the ipsilateral lung usually provides sufficient working space for visualization and instrument manipulation.

To address the significant morbidity that can occur following trocar injury to a vascular structure or bowel, several innovative features have been introduced. Trocars with optical viewing capability during insertion, use of a fascial- or tissue-separating blunt tip, threaded cannulas placed with a twisting motion, or combinations thereof, are now widely used. Even with the use of optical trocars, injuries still occur,[9,12] and, despite any and all of the safety features mentioned above, 15% to 22% of all laparoscopic trocar injuries occur during the placement of secondary trocars, with the trocar entry under direct visualization.[13–15] Thus, one must be familiar with proper trocar placement technique and be cognizant of structures immediately beneath the entry site. This requirement is especially true in humans, who are anatomically flattened in the dorsal-ventral plane. Our veterinary patients, although flattened in a lateral plane such that the aorta and other large vessels are deeper, are still subject to injury, particularly smaller patients.

Trocars may be single-patient use, reusable, or a hybrid, providing for easy replacement of components that wear easily, such as the sharp obturator tip. Reusable trocars, or trocars with reusable components may be the most economical alternative for veterinary clinical practice, as insurance reimbursement for single-patient devices

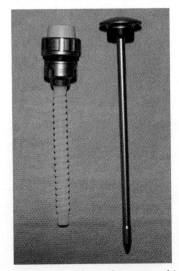

Fig. 13. A flexible, reusable, trocar with a blunt obturator, which is ideal for thoracoscopic applications. The pliability of the cannula is less traumatic to anatomic structures immediately adjacent to the cannula. A rigid cannula is preferred for protecting the rigid scope if placed between the ribs.

available in human medicine is largely unavailable in veterinary practice. Many veterinary practitioners currently performing minimally invasive procedures have developed their own internal protocols for reprocessing and sterilizing laparoscopic instrumentation, including trocars. Affiliation with a local hospital, human surgeons and surgical team members who are clients, and online auction forums have also enabled many veterinary practitioners to acquire minimally invasive equipment economically. Provided strict, academic principles of surgery and asepsis are followed, creativity within these constraints has enabled practitioners to acquire the necessary equipment for performing minimally invasive surgery, including the designing and making of devices themselves.

New trocars are available that provide for the introduction of multiple instruments through a single port, allowing procedures to be performed with less morbidity. For example, instead of placing multiple ports through the abdominal wall as the authors typically do in laparoscopic surgery, a single port can be placed through the umbilicus to accommodate multiple instruments simultaneously. This technique is being called natural orifice transumbilical surgery (NOTUS). An example of key, enabling innovation in this area is an access port in which the valves have been removed and "Air-Seal" technology seals the device, no matter how many instruments are inserted (AirSeal, SurgiQuest Inc, Orange, CT, USA). This new, single puncture approach has led to new developments in hand instruments that articulate by way of simple wrist motion and enable the surgeon to perform many tasks without the chopsticking one would expect to encounter from being deployed coaxially through a single trocar. Chopsticking is the term that describes the interference that can occur between instruments when they are deployed coaxially through a common channel or within close proximity to one another As procedures become more advanced, additional innovative features are being incorporated into trocar design, including the use of magnetic forces in the trocar which guide the various tips, or end-effectors, to the trocar cannula lumen and allow the surgeons to exchange laparoscopic instruments without looking away from the video monitor.

HAND INSTRUMENTS

A selection of laparoscopic hand instruments should be available that is complementary to that used in identical open procedures. The end-effectors of laparoscopic instruments are identical to their conventional counterparts except that the instrument is much longer (**Fig. 14**). In fact, the greatest differences between laparoscopic instruments and conventional instruments are length and the resultant loss of tactile feedback. Laparoscopic instrumentation may come with a more traditional pistol grip handle configuration, which may or may not be ratcheted, or an in-line configuration (**Figs. 15** and **16**). The advantage of the pistol-grip configuration is that the instrument may feel more stable in the hand, but this is highly dependent on the user's preferences. An in-line handle is more readily amenable to rotation of the instrument around its long axis, and is therefore commonly employed in needle holders for laparoscopic suturing.

Characteristics of the instruments in general that one must consider for performing a given procedure are: length; the diameter of the instrument (3 mm, 5 mm, 10 mm being the most commonly used); the ability to rotate the shaft and end-effector; the ability to apply energy (monopolar or bipolar, and so forth); presence of a ratcheting mechanism allowing the instrument to be locked on the tissue; whether the device is for single-patient use or is reusable; and whether the device is single- or double-action. A single-action end-effector simply implies that only one of the opposing

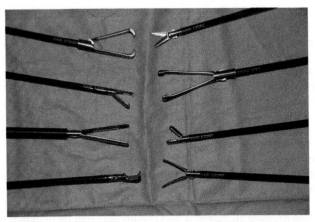

Fig. 14. Photo depicting a variety of end-effectors on laparoscopic instruments.

jaws of the instrument moves when the handle is open and closed, whereas in double-action instruments both of the opposing jaws of the instrument move. Logically, a double-action instrument, for example a curved Kelly dissector, would be preferable for fine dissection, as it would most closely mimic the action of a conventional instrument used in the same manner during an open procedure.

Instrumentation is available that affords the surgeon a large degree of articulation at the end-effector, allowing the instrument to interact with the tissue from various angles of approach without having to place additional trocars. Such modifications provide a means for multiple articulating instruments to be placed through a single trocar for access to a target site and used by the operator without chopsticking as described previously (RealHand HD Instruments, Novare Surgical Systems, Cupertino, CA, USA, and Autonomy Laparo-Angle Instrumentation, Cambridge Endo, Framingham, MA, USA).

One of the most important disadvantages to overcome in the use of laparoscopic instrumentation is the loss of tactile feedback. The same principles of atraumatic tissue handling apply to laparoscopic instrumentation. For example, one would not apply an Allis tissue clamp to a loop of bowel unless it was to be resected, but, with the loss of tactile feedback, a laparoscopic instrument that is designed to be atraumatic could cause serious injury if misused.

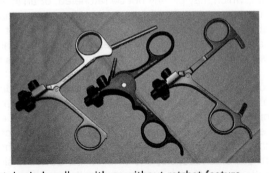

Fig. 15. Various pistol-grip handles, with or without ratchet feature.

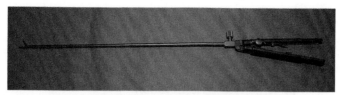

Fig. 16. Laparoscopic needle driver with in-line handle, which facilitates rotation of the instrument about the long axis.

Laparoscopic scissors are also available in many configurations, depending on the need, can be disposable or reusable, and are often equipped for the application of energy such as monopolar or bipolar cautery. The use of electrocautery on scissors can dramatically decrease the blade life. The disadvantage of reusable scissors is the need for periodic sharpening; however, disposable laparoscopic scissors may be less economical depending on the resources of the operator.

Many other specialized instruments are available, including combination devices such as a suction/flush/monopolar dissection probe (**Fig. 17**). Cottonoid dissectors are useful in performing blunt dissection of loose areolar tissues (**Fig. 18**).

There are several vessel sealing devices that enable the surgeon to transect large vascularized pedicles without the need for vascular clips or suture-based methodologies. Many of these devices will effectively seal vessels up to 3 to 7 mm in diameter. Examples include the EnSeal (SurgRx Inc, Redwood City, CA, USA), Ligasure devices (Valleylab, Boulder, CO, USA) and Harmonic devices (Ethicon Endo-Surgery, Cincinnati, OH, USA). They enable laparoscopic ovariohysterectomy or ovariectomy with relative ease in small or larger patients. Disadvantages are cost and that they are designed for single-patient use. More economical alternatives for control of large vascular structures are available, such as the use of pretied suture loops or intracorporeal or extracorporeal techniques, which can be efficient with practice.

Extraction of tissue can be accomplished through the use of specialized retrieval bags deployed through a trocar cannula. These devices may be used to isolate the tissues of the body wall from the potential seeding of metastases when suspect neoplastic tissues are being removed, as portal site metastasis has been reported in the literature.[16] For larger tissues that will not fit through a trocar cannula, a tissue morcellator can be used, which enables the tissue to be sectioned into smaller pieces intracorporeally and then extracted in piecemeal fashion. Alternatively, the trocar incision may be enlarged to accommodate extraction of the tissue, or a portion of the procedure may be completed in a conventional or laparoscopic-assisted manner.

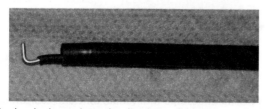

Fig. 17. A monopolar hook electrode at the distal tip of a laparoscopic flush/suction probe.

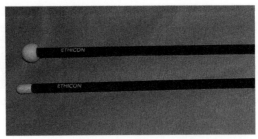

Fig.18. Single-use cottonoid dissectors are available in various sizes and shapes for performing blunt dissection.

FLEXIBLE ENDOSCOPY
Flexible Endoscopes

Flexible endoscopes are most useful when the operator needs to navigate more complex anatomy, typically within the lumen of an organ. The gastroscope is the most versatile flexible endoscope in veterinary practice, with potential applications in small and large animals for GI, respiratory, and urinary tract procedures, depending on patient size. Typically, gastroscopes range from 8 to 10 mm in diameter. The manual controls and working-channel opening are incorporated into a handpiece (**Fig. 19**) from which the insertion tube extends. The insertion tube enters the patient, and its length and diameter are essentially determined by the intended use(s) of the endoscope. The umbilical cord extends from the handpiece, and plugs into the light source. It may also have fittings for insufflation, irrigation, and suction. A pressure-compensation valve may be present on the distal end of the umbilical cord and is used for leak testing. This valve also serves to open the internal environment of the endoscope during high-pressure events, such as ethylene oxide sterilization or air cargo transport. The insufflation and irrigation components are driven by an air pump, which may be a separate unit, or, in some systems, integrated into the light source. Irrigation fluid must be distilled (or demineralized) to prevent mineral deposits from blocking the channel. Standard suction may be attached to the suction connector on the handpiece. Insufflation is required to distend the walls of the viscus or luminal structure(s) to optimize visualization. Irrigation clears the viewing lens of the

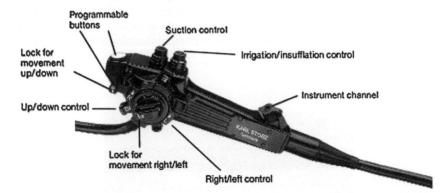

Fig.19. Handpiece of flexible endoscope with various controls. (*Courtesy of* Karl Storz GmbH & Co. KG, Tuttlingen, Germany.)

scope of blood, fog, or other debris. Suction clears fluid(s) and tempers the amount of insufflation. Controls for these features are located on the handpiece.

Most flexible endoscopes have a working (instrument) channel able to accommodate several devices, such as a cytology brush, biopsy forceps, foreign body retrieval forceps, and so forth. Using the instrument channel significantly reduces or eliminates suction capability, as the instrument channel is the suction channel as well. It is also worth mentioning that instruments inserted through the working channel must be deflected in a position to avoid damaging the inner lining of the channel. The diameter of the working channel should be a minimum of 2 mm to procure biopsy samples of diagnostic quality.[17]

Gentle deflection of the endoscope is controlled by knobs on the handpiece. Rotation of these knobs results in lengthening or shortening of cables that run the length of the insertion tube to the bendable portion of the scope. Control of up and down deflection of the tip is accomplished by rotating the larger outer knob, and control of left and right deflection by rotation of the smaller inner knob (**Fig. 19**). Each of the knobs is equipped with a locking lever, allowing the operator to lock the tip in any position. For most gastroscopes, maximal deflection is in the up position and should be a minimum of 180°. Deflection in each of the other three planes should be at least 90°. Smaller flexible endoscopes, which have a working channel, often have only two-way tip deflection.

For GI applications, sterility of the flexible scope is less critical. However, for respiratory and urinary applications, the endoscope should be sterilized. Because of the environment in which flexible endoscopes are used, it is of utmost importance that they be watertight so that the inner components are not damaged by corrosion or staining of fiberoptic bundles, which can weaken them and cause them to break prematurely. Leak testing of flexible endoscopes should be performed before and after every procedure. Small leaks, if identified early, are reparable.

When considering a flexible endoscope for purchase, there are many considerations, one of the most important of which is size. For small animal practice, flexible endoscopes with a diameter less than 10 mm and longer than 125 cm are most useful, although greater length is required for duodenoscopy in large dogs.[18] Smaller-diameter endoscopes, ranging from 55 to 100 cm in length, are available for use in the respiratory and urinary tracts, and are also available in extended lengths for bronchoscopy and cystoscopy in large dogs.

Optical quality and whether it is sufficient to enable the practitioner to perform the desired tasks are additional considerations. The ability of the endoscope to adequately illuminate the desired area(s) is also a critical factor. These traits are best evaluated in a side-by-side comparison; what can be visualized from within a large, hollow, insufflated viscus may be different from what one is able to see in a simple table-top demonstration.

Before acquiring any endoscopic equipment, ensure that the vendor is able to provide adequate turn-around time for repairs, and that loaner equipment is available so that your practice is not impacted significantly when or if repairs or service are required.

Fiberscope Versus Video-Endoscope

A fiberscope or fiberoptic endoscope and a video-endoscope comprise the two types of flexible endoscopes available. Both use a fiberoptic bundle to conduct light for illuminating the target area, but they differ in how the image is transmitted and displayed on the video monitor. A fiberscope conducts the image by way of a fiberoptic bundle from a lens at the tip of the endoscope to the lens at the eyepiece. A video camera is attached for transmitting the image to the video monitor. With a video-endoscope, a CCD sensor (chip) is positioned behind the objective lens at the distal tip of the endoscope (**Fig. 20**), and the image is conducted electronically along the length of the endoscope to a video processor, and ultimately to a viewing monitor.

The quality of a fiberoptic image is directly related to the number and size of optical fibers, the quality with which they are bound, and the quality of the lenses at the proximal and distal ends of the fiberoptic imaging bundle. If the fibers are large, the image may have a pixilated, or a honeycomb, appearance. Broken fibers will result in dark spots in the image due to loss of transmission of light, as described for evaluating light-guide cables for laparoscopic evaluations. The image resolution of a fiberscope is inferior to that of a video-endoscope.

Most veterinary practitioners use fiberscopes, because the detachable video camera can be used with so many other endoscopes, thereby expanding the endoscopic capabilities of the practice without investing in more costly video-endoscopes.

Instrumentation

In addition to the cytology brushes, biopsy forceps, and foreign-body graspers mentioned previously, there is a significant number of other instruments available to the practitioner, including stone retrieval baskets, bronchoalveolar lavage tubing, polypectomy snares, monopolar needle knife, scissors, injection/apiration needles, and laser fibers (**Fig. 21**). One may elect to use reusable or disposable instruments; however, reusable instruments, although more expensive at the outset, are more economical over the long term, if cared for properly. Proper care of reusable instruments includes careful cleaning, lubricating, and storing, in accordance with the manufacturer's guidelines.

CARE AND CLEANING OF ENDOSCOPIC EQUIPMENT AND COMPONENTS

Following the manufacturer's recommendations for cleaning, maintaining, sterilizing, and storing endoscopic equipment is the best approach to maximize longevity of endoscopic equipment, instruments, and components. For new equipment, not doing so may void the warranty and result in significant expense to the practitioner.

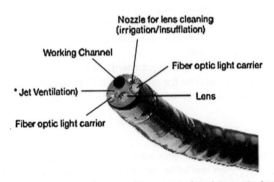

Fig. 20. The distal end of a video-endoscope. (*Courtesy of* Karl Storz GmbH & Co. KG, Tuttlingen, Germany.)

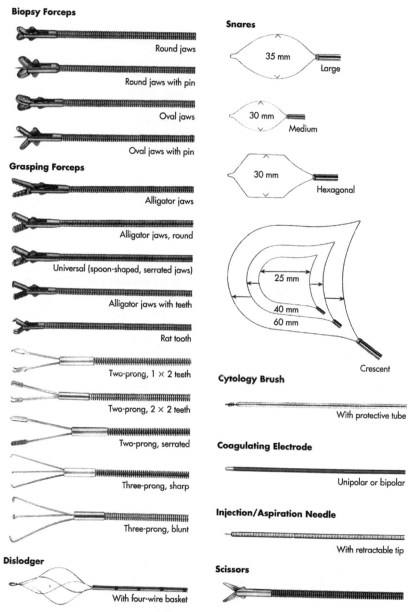

Fig. 21. Various end-effectors of flexible endoscopic instruments. (*From* Tams T. Small animal endoscopy. Philadelphia: Elsevier, 1998; with permission.)

Particular attention should be paid to whether the component/equipment is submersible for cleaning/sterilizing, or whether it is autoclavable, or gas sterilizable. As mentioned previously, a pressure compensation cap must be used when gas sterilizing a flexible endoscope.

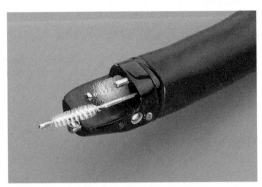

Fig. 22. Cleaning brushes protruding from a flexible endoscope with two working channels. (*Courtesy of* Karl Storz GmbH & Co. KG, Tuttlingen, Germany.)

Generally speaking, all instrumentation should be cleaned immediately after use with brushes specifically designed for the respective instruments and scopes (**Fig. 22**). Hand instruments and trocars should be taken apart during cleaning and sterilizing to ensure all component parts are cleaned and exposed to the sterilizing agent/process. Cleaning solutions should be of a neutral pH and any water used for flushing component parts, working channels, or dilution of cleaning agents should be distilled or demineralized.

Specialized trays are available for storing and sterilizing endoscopic instruments (**Fig. 23**). Flexible scopes should be stored in a hanging position when not in use, to enable drainage of residual fluid from the luminal channels and to prevent undue cyclic stress on fiberoptic elements, which might otherwise occur if stored in a coiled fashion for extended periods.

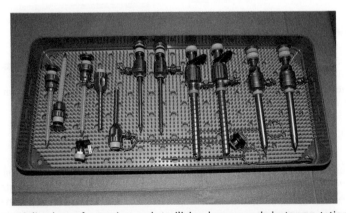

Fig. 23. A specialized tray for storing and sterilizing laparoscopic instrumentation.

REFERENCES

1. Online Health Library. University of Chicago Medical Center. 11-12-2008. 12-11-2008.
2. Devitt CM, Cox RE, Hailey JJ. Duration, complications, stress, and pain of open ovariohysterectomy versus a simple method of laparoscopic-assisted ovariohysterectomy in dogs. J Am Vet Med Assoc 2005;227(6):921–7.
3. Marcovich R, Williams AL, Seifman BD, et al. A canine model to assess the biochemical stress response to laparoscopic and open surgery. J Endourol 2001;15(10):1005–8.
4. Naitoh T, Garcia-Ruiz A, Vladisavljevic A, et al. Gastrointestinal transit and stress response after laparoscopic vs conventional distal pancreatectomy in the canine model. Surg Endosc 2002;16(11):1627–30.
5. Walsh PJ, Remedios AM, Ferguson JF, et al. Thoracoscopic versus open partial pericardectomy in dogs: comparison of postoperative pain and morbidity. Vet Surg 1999;28(6):472–9.
6. Freeman LJ. Operating room setup, equipment, and instrumentation. In: Freeman LJ, editor. Veterinary endosurgery. 1st edition. St. Louis (MO): Mosby; 1999. p. 3–23.
7. Yin L, Witten CM, Neidelman SM. Letter to manufacturers of laparoscopic trocars. FDA, Center for Devices and Radiologic Health, Rockville (MD), 1996.
8. Champault G, Cazacu F, Taffinder N. Serious trocar accidents in laparoscopic surgery: a French survey of 103,852 operations. Surg Laparosc Endosc 1996; 6(5):367–70.
9. Corson SL, Chandler JG, Way LW. Survey of laparoscopic entry injuries provoking litigation. J Am Assoc Gynecol Laparosc 2001;8(3):341–7.
10. HarkkiSiren P, Kurki T. A nationwide analysis of laparoscopic complications. Obstet Gynecol 1997;89(1):108–12.
11. Kazemier G, Hazebroek EJ, Lange JF, et al. Needle and trocar injury during laparoscopic surgery in Japan. Surg Endosc 1999;13(2):194.
12. Sharp HT, Dodson MK, Draper ML, et al. Complications associated with optical-access laparoscopic trocars. Obstet Gynecol 2002;99(4):553–5.
13. Hashizume M, Sugimachi K. Needle and trocar injury during laparoscopic surgery in Japan. Surg Endosc 1997;11(12):1198–201.
14. Chapron C, Pierre F, Harchaoui Y, et al. Gastrointestinal injuries during gynaecological laparoscopy. Humanit Rep 1999;14(2):333–7.
15. Yuzpe AA. Pneumoperitoneum needle and trocar injuries in laparoscopy - a survey on possible contributing factors and prevention. J Reprod Med 1990;35(5): 485–90.
16. Brisson BA, Reggeti F, Bienzle D. Portal site metastasis of invasive mesothelioma after diagnostic thoracoscopy in a dog. J Am Vet Med Assoc 2006;229(6):980–3.
17. Chamness CJ. Instrumentation. In: Lhermette P, Sobel D, editors. BSAVA manual of canine and feline endoscopy and endosurgery. 1st edition. Gloucester (England): British Small Animal Veterinary Association; 2008. p. 11–30.
18. Chamness CJ. Introduction to veterinary endoscopy and endoscopic instrumentation. In: McCarthy TC, editor. Veterinary endoscopy. 1st edition. Missouri: Elsevier Saunders; 2005. p. 1–20.

Anesthesia for Endoscopy in Small Animals

Ann B. Weil, MS, DVM

KEYWORDS

- Anesthesia • Endoscopy • Small animals • Monitoring
- Drug recommendations

Endoscopy is the process of looking inside the body by inserting a rigid or flexible tube into the body and examining an image of the interior of an organ or cavity. An additional instrument may be inserted to take a tissue biopsy or retrieve foreign objects. It is considered a minimally invasive diagnostic or medical procedure in animals, but most endoscopic procedures in dogs and cats will require general anesthesia nevertheless. Endoscopic procedures are often used to examine the respiratory system (laryngoscopy/tracheoscopy/bronchoscopy), gastrointestinal (GI) system (upper and lower GI endoscopy), thoracic cavity (thoracoscopy), abdomen (laparoscopy), urinary tract (cystoscopy), or joints (arthroscopy). Many of the potential complications of endoscopic procedures are related to general anesthesia.[1] Some endoscopic procedures require special anesthetic considerations, whereas some (arthroscopy, cystoscopy) tend to be more straightforward. A thorough understanding of the physiologic changes produced by various endoscopic procedures is necessary to properly support an anesthetized patient. Many endoscopic procedures require the use of an insufflation gas to facilitate visualization, with resulting physiologic changes to the patient. Body position of the patient during the procedure may also have profound effects on the cardiovascular and respiratory systems. A complete knowledge of all anesthetics and adjunctive drugs is necessary to support patient care.

GENERAL CONSIDERATIONS

Patients undergoing general anesthesia should have food withheld for 12 hours before the procedure. The patient should have access to water up to an hour before the start of general anesthesia. Pediatric patients and other patients at risk for hypoglycemia should have a shorter fasting period. Baseline data include a complete blood count (CBC), chemistry panel with electrolytes, and urinalysis. Other ancillary tests that may be considered include thoracic and abdominal radiographs, ECG,

---

Department of Veterinary Clinical Sciences, School of Veterinary Medicine Purdue University, 625 Harrison Street, West Lafayette, IN 47907, USA
E-mail address: aweil@purdue.edu

Vet Clin Small Anim 39 (2009) 839–848
doi:10.1016/j.cvsm.2009.05.008
0195-5616/09/$ – see front matter © 2009 Elsevier Inc. All rights reserved.

echocardiogram, and blood gas analysis, depending on the body systems affected and the planned procedure.

Drug choices should be individualized. Premedication tranquilizers/sedatives such as acepromazine or benzodiazepines help calm patients before catheter placement and improve recovery conditions. Opioids will add analgesia and sedation. The use of premedications will reduce the amount of injectable and inhalant anesthetics needed by the patient, thus improving cardiovascular performance. Anticholinergics (atropine, glycopyrrolate) should be used when patients require an increase in heart rate; they can counteract the increase in vagal tone produced by administered drugs (opioids) or procedure (cystoscopy). Injectable anesthetics include propofol, thiopental, ketamine, or etomidate. Isoflurane or sevoflurane may be used as a maintenance inhalant agent. **Table 1** lists sample protocols for various endoscopic procedures. Specific drug concerns are discussed in each section.

Monitoring of the anesthetized patient undergoing a minimally invasive procedure is just as important as if they were undergoing major surgery. Invasive or noninvasive blood pressure measurement, pulse oximetry, capnometry, and ECG can be useful for assessing and maintaining normal physiologic parameters in the anesthetized patient. Mean arterial pressure should be maintained higher than 60 mmHg in dogs and cats. End-tidal CO_2 should be between 35 and 45 mmHg and SpO_2 greater than 95%. Crystalloid fluids should be administered to patients undergoing inhalant anesthesia for minimally invasive procedures, as inhalant anesthetics cause vasodilation and decreased venous return, regardless of the anticipated amount of blood loss. Crystalloid fluids are generally administered at a rate of 10 mL/kg/h unless the patient is hypoproteinemic, has cardiac disease, anuria, and so forth. Patients that are dehydrated before the procedure should have their volume deficit corrected before general anesthesia.[2] Some patients may benefit from the administration of colloids while undergoing the procedure.

LARYNGOSCOPY/TRACHEOSCOPY

Many patients undergoing this diagnostic procedure will have signs of obstructive upper airway disease. They are dyspneic and easily stressed. Thoracic radiographs should be added to the minimum database if the images can be obtained without excessive stress to the patient. Evaluation of laryngeal function is most frequently done under a light plane of general anesthesia.[3] A variety of injectable anesthetics have been used. All sedative drugs and deeper planes of anesthesia tend to diminish arytenoid function with much individual variation. The perfect technique of general anesthesia for laryngeal function evaluation has yet to be established, as the depth of anesthesia must be sufficient enough to open the jaw and protect the examiner and equipment, yet still maintain arytenoid cartilage movement for evaluation. False-positive examinations can occur with most sedatives and anesthetic combinations.

Preoxygenation of the patient by way of an oxygen mask or flow-by oxygen with the breathing circuit is helpful. Two to 3 L/min of oxygen should be given for 5 minutes immediately before drug administration. This procedure allows increased time for examination of the airway before the patient desaturates. A variety of injectable anesthetic protocols have been evaluated. One study showed that arytenoid motion at recovery was significantly greater with thiopental compared with propofol alone, acepromazine with thiopental or propofol, and ketamine and diazepam.[4] This is comparable with what has been shown in people, in whom propofol has been reported to have a more detrimental effect on vocal cord motion than thiopental.[5] Another study did not show any difference between thiopental, propofol, or diazepam-ketamine

Table 1
Sample anesthetic protocols for selected endoscopic procedures.

1. Bronchoscopy

 Premedication: acepromazine (0.02 mg/kg)

 Induction: propofol 6 mg/kg IV to effect

 Maintain: isoflurane or sevoflurane if endotracheal (ET) tube >7

  Propofol CRI (0.15–0.4 mg/kg/min) or intermittent bolus

 Postprocedure: oxygen therapy

2. Upper GI endoscopy

 Premedication:

  Acepromazine (0.02 mg/kg) or midazolam (0.1–0.2 mg/kg)

  Butorphanol (0.2 mg/kg) or hydromorphone (0.05–0.1 mg/kg) or buprenorphine
  (0.005–0.015 mg/kg)

 Induction: propofol 6 mg/kg IV to effect or ketamine (5 mg/kg)/diazepam (0.2 mg/kg)

 Maintain: isoflurane or sevoflurane

 Postprocedure: repeat opioid

3. Rhinoscopy

 Premedication: acepromazine (0.02 mg/kg) or dexmedetomidine (0.0025–0.005 mg/kg) or
 midazolam (0.1–0.2 mg/kg) IM or subcutaneous (SC)

 Hydromorphone (0.1 mg/kg) or morphine (0.5 mg/kg) IM

 Induction: propofol 6 mg/kg IV to effect or ketamine (5 mg/kg)/diazepam (0.2 mg/kg)

 Maintain: isoflurane or sevoflurane

 Intraop: fentanyl 1–3 μg/kg bolus

  Infraorbital block: lidocaine 0.25–0.5 mL

 Postprocedure: repeat opioid, give additional acepromazine or dexmedetomidine as needed
 for sedation

4. Laparoscopy or thoracoscopy

 Premedication: acepromazine (0.01–0.02 mg/kg) or midazolam (0.1–0.2 mg/kg)

 Opioids:

  Hydromorphone (0.05–0.1 mg/kg) IM or IV

  Morphine (0.25–0.5 mg/kg) IM

  Fentanyl (1–3 μg/kg bolus, then 5–10 μg/kg CRI)

  Buprenorphine (0.01 mg/kg)

  Butorphanol (0.2–0.4 mg/kg)

 Induction:

  Propofol (6 mg/kg) IV to effect

  Diazepam/ketamine (0.2 mg/kg)/(5 mg/kg) IV

  Diazepam/etomidate (0.2 mg/kg)/(1–2 mg/kg) IV to effect

 Maintenance:

  Isoflurane

  Sevoflurane

 Post procedure:

  Repeat opioid

  Administer regional anesthesia: lidocaine patch application

when evaluating laryngeal function in dogs premedicated with butorphanol and glyco-pyrrolate.[6] Other disease conditions of the patient should be taken into consideration before the final selection of anesthetic agent, as well as the conditions under which the examiner is accustomed to doing the evaluation. It is helpful for an assistant to announce inspiration by the patient while evaluating arytenoid abduction. Propofol may be administered at 6 mg/kg intravenously (IV) or thiopental at 12 mg/kg to good effect. Administration of supplemental oxygen during the examination is useful, as is pulse oximetry to monitor oxygen saturation. Some authors recommend doxap-ram administration (2–5 mg/kg IV) at the end of the examination to stimulate more vigorous respiratory movements and eliminate false positives.[4]

Although general anesthesia is most frequently used for laryngoscopy and laryngeal function evaluation, a transnasal approach under sedation has been used to diagnose laryngeal paralysis in large breed dogs.[7] An opioid analgesic and acepromazine were given to each animal intramuscularly (IM) and lidocaine applied topically to the left nasal passage 30 minutes after sedation, to facilitate passage of the endoscope.

General anesthesia is used for tracheoscopy and bronchoscopy in animals to mini-mize laryngospasm and coughing and protect the endoscope. Tracheoscopy/bron-choscopy is performed without an endotracheal tube in small patients or with the endotracheal tube in patients with sufficient tracheal diameter (size 7 or 8 endotra-cheal tube). Inhalant anesthesia can be used to maintain the patient during bronchos-copy if the patient is large enough for an endotracheal tube, using a special T-shaped adapter to accommodate the scope as well as administer oxygen and anesthetic gas.[8] There should be sufficient room inside the endotracheal tube for exhalation of gases without resistance.

Injectable anesthetics can be used to maintain anesthesia in patients with small tracheal diameter, whereas oxygen is administered through the scope or through a catheter placed beside the scope if there is sufficient room. A variety of injectable protocols may be used, depending on the patient condition. In general, an injectable protocol that has minimal cardiovascular effects and allows rapid recovery is prefer-able, as many patients undergoing bronchoscopy have significant respiratory impair-ment. Short-acting opioids can be used for premedication, such as fentanyl or butorphanol. Butorphanol is a potent cough suppressant. Acepromazine has little respiratory depression and is useful at low doses to calm patients with upper respira-tory disease. Propofol has little accumulative effect[9] and can be administered in inter-mittent boluses or by constant rate infusion (CRI) to maintain anesthesia. The use of anticholinergics to dry up small airways is no longer recommended. Oxygen supple-mentation post tracheoscopy or bronchoscopy is important to support patients through the recovery period until airway reflexes are normal.

Oxygen saturation should be monitored by pulse oximetry throughout the procedure, with the goal of maintaining saturation greater than 95%. Mean arterial blood pressure should be greater than 60 mmHg. Administration of balanced, isotonic crystalloid fluids should be used with inhalant anesthesia and propofol CRI of moderate duration.

UPPER GASTROINTESTINAL ENDOSCOPY

Anesthetic drugs may alter intestinal motility, sphincter function, and promote vomit-ing. Upper GI endoscopy is impossible to perform without general anesthesia in dogs and cats. The esophagus, stomach, and upper duodenum can be visualized and a biopsy taken if warranted. If the patient has experienced prolonged vomiting, the animal should be carefully examined for dehydration or electrolyte disturbances. Volume depletion and electrolyte imbalance should be corrected before general anesthesia. The animal may be sedated with a mild tranquilizer like acepromazine if not dehydrated. Full μ opioid agonists like morphine, oxymorphone, or hydromorphone may promote vomiting if administered IM. Drugs that potentiate vomiting should be avoided in cases of esophageal or gastric foreign bodies. κ opioid agonists such as butorphanol are less likely to promote vomiting. The animal should be induced with an injectable anesthetic and intubated quickly to avoid aspiration. Propofol, thiopental, ketamine, or etomidate may be used for this purpose, depending on the rest of the animal's condition. The patient may be maintained on inhalants after intubation. An appropriately inflated endotracheal tube cuff should be maintained at all times to avoid inadvertent aspiration of fluid during the procedure.

Balanced, isotonic crystalloid fluids (such as Normosol-R [Norm-R] or lactated Ringer's solution [LRS]) administered at 10 mL/kg/h should be used for patients with normal oncotic pressure and plasma proteins. Hypoproteinemic patients may benefit from colloid administration. Plasma or hetastarch can be used to assist in maintaining sufficient oncotic pressure. Hetastarch can be used at a rate of 5 mL/kg/h along with crystalloid fluid administration during the procedure. Care must be taken to avoid fluid overload.

Insufflation of the stomach with air must be carefully monitored to avoid overinflation and attendant cardiovascular and respiratory compromise.[10] Pulse oximetry, blood pressure, and capnometry are helpful to monitor anesthesia in these patients. Frequently respiration must be supported with intermittent positive pressure ventilation if abdominal pressure is increased. The size of the stomach should be continuously monitored during gastroscopy.

Care must be taken to avoid aspiration of gastric contents. The endotracheal tube cuff should be properly inflated on intubation and maintained throughout the procedure. The cuff should not be deflated until the patient is extubated, ensuring that the patient can swallow and the airway is protected.

The cardiac and pyloric sphincters can impede endoscopy.[11] Comparison of premedication with atropine, glycopyrrolate, morphine, meperidine, acepromazine, and saline before general anesthesia for gastroduodenoscopy in dogs resulted in more difficulty in entering the pyloric sphincter when a combination of morphine and atropine was used.[12] This has led to the suggestion that all full μ opioid agonists be avoided when duodenoscopy is performed. The use of atropine in dogs as a premedication does not facilitate duodenal intubation and may inhibit it.[13] α2 agonists such as medetomidine do not hinder the passage of the endoscope through the pylorus in dogs, although vomiting may be an issue in some patients.[14]

More recent work has evaluated the effects of various premedications on ease of duodenoscopy in the cat.[15] Their results suggest that hydromorphone (a full μ opioid agonist), glycopyrrolate (anticholinergic), medetomidine (α2 agonist), or butorphanol (agonist antagonist opioid) are all satisfactory for use as a premedication before gastroduodenoscopy in the cat.

Experienced clinicians may not have any difficulty passing the endoscope into the duodenum, despite the anesthetic protocol used. Butorphanol may be used without difficulty and has the additional benefit of not inducing as much vomiting as a full μ agonist when used as a premedication. Its short duration is helpful in avoiding excessive post anesthetic sedation.

COLONOSCOPY

Colonoscopy is often performed in patients with signs of large bowel or rectal disease.[16] To adequately visualize the colonic mucosa, the bowel is prepared for the procedure with food withdrawal, administration of a GI lavage solution (eg, Go-LYTELY, Braintree Laboratories, Braintree, Massachusetts) and a series of enemas.[16] This preparation can cause dehydration in some patients. Careful evaluation should be performed to ensure adequate hydration before general anesthesia. Volume deficits should be corrected before general anesthesia with IV administration of crystalloid fluids.

Complications associated with colonoscopy are reported to be rare in dogs, with minor and major complications developing in 30 out of 355 procedures (8.5%).[17] Minor complications were most frequently associated with vomiting of GoLYTELY. Anesthetic complications such as bradycardia that resolved after the anesthetic episode were also reported under minor complications. Major complications may also be associated with general anesthesia. Aspiration of vomited GoLYTELY was responsible for mortality of one patient in the study and has been reported in humans.[16,18] Care must be taken to protect the airway during the procedure.

RHINOSCOPY

Rhinoscopy patients need to have good analgesia in their anesthetic protocol, as the procedure requires a surgical plane of anesthesia.[19] A full μ opioid agonist such as hydromorphone, morphine, or oxymorphone can be administered as part of the premedication in addition to a tranquilizer such as acepromazine or an α2 sedative. Short-acting potent opioids such as fentanyl can be bolused intravenously before biopsy to prevent excessively high vaporizer settings. Regional anesthetic techniques such as infraorbital blocks with lidocaine, mepivicaine, or bupivicaine will also improve patient comfort. Postprocedure bleeding can be minimized if the patient is well sedated after biopsies are taken, as excessive head shaking and activity can lead to continued bleeding and increased irritation of the area.

The endotracheal cuff should be properly inflated before rhinoscopy and the procedure halted any time there is a concern about the cuff. It can be helpful to extubate the patient with the cuff partially inflated to assist in clearing blood from the airway if it has not been packed before beginning the procedure.

LAPAROSCOPY

Laparoscopic noninvasive surgery has become common as more procedures are attempted in a noninvasive fashion. To perform this type of surgery, a pneumoperitoneum is established to allow room to place the trocar and cannula assemblies safely and improve visualization.[1] Several gases have been used to insufflate the abdomen: carbon dioxide, nitrous oxide, or room air. Carbon dioxide is most frequently chosen as the insufflation gas for laparoscopy.[20] The use of medical air has increased potential for air embolism and increased potential to support combustion if electrocautery is used. Carbon dioxide is able to diffuse across the peritoneal cavity and enter the blood stream, whereby it stimulates the sympathetic nervous system to release endogenous catecholamines. Higher levels of arterial CO_2 tend to increase heart rate, blood pressure, and cardiac output. Excessively high levels of CO_2 will lead to narcosis, arrhythmia, acidemia, and myocardial depression. Nitrous oxide does not alter the patient's acid-base status.

Regardless of the type of gas used, insufflation of gas increases intraabdominal pressure (IAP) in the patient, with the potential to cause decreased tidal volume and hypoventilation. Functional residual capacity and lung compliance decrease during general anesthesia.[21,22] The increase in IAP from gas insufflation causes cranial displacement of the diaphragm. All of these factors contribute to the need for increased ventilation support for the anesthetized patient undergoing laparoscopy. Depression of ventilation increases with increasing IAP and IAP less than 20 mmHg is recommended.[23]

Increased IAP also leads to decreased venous return and a reduction in cardiac output. Tissue blood flow may be compromised with increased IAP as elevated IAPs are associated with decreased hepatic blood flow and oliguria.[24] Anesthetic conditions for the patient will be improved by using the least amount of IAP necessary to complete the procedure.

Changes in body position have the potential to adversely affect the anesthetized patient, especially if coupled with abdominal insufflation. Inhalant anesthetics alter the baroreflex, leading to a depressed reflex control of circulation in response to changes in body posture.[24–26] Head down tilt of a dorsally recumbent patient (Trendelenburg position) allows for better exposure of the caudal organs in the operative field. Reverse Trendelenburg position (head up and dorsally recumbent) is used if improved exposure of cranial organs is desired. The head down tilt position has more effect on respiratory and cardiovascular mechanics, leading to decreases in minute ventilation and cardiac output, amongst other things. Mean arterial pressure may increase. The head up tilt position will also affect cardiovascular mechanics, leading to reflex vasoconstriction, and increased heart rate and arterial blood pressure in dogs.[27]

Excellent monitoring of the anesthetized patient undergoing laparoscopy is essential. Increased IAP results in hypoventilation, so the use of a mechanical ventilator is helpful to provide pulmonary support as normocapnia should be a monitoring goal. If CO_2 is the insufflation gas used, absorption of CO_2 across the peritoneal membrane will lead to higher $PaCO_2$, regardless of the respiratory status of the patient. End-tidal CO_2 monitoring and pulse oximetry will provide continuous monitoring of the respiratory system. Invasive blood pressure monitoring is warranted in more critical patients undergoing laparoscopy, whereas noninvasive methods (Doppler or oscillometric cuff-based monitors) can be used in healthy patients undergoing elective laparoscopic procedures. Arterial catheter placement will allow easier sampling for blood gas analysis if CO_2 is the insufflation gas. Abdominal insufflation must be monitored and the rule of 15s is a good general guideline: no more than 15 mmHg IAP or 15 degrees of tilt.[24]

General anesthesia is most frequently used for laparoscopic procedures in small animals, but it is important to consider the increased stress to the patient of abdominal insufflation and tilted body posture. These effects are aggravated by general anesthesia. A recent study compared the cardiopulmonary effects of laparoscopic-assisted jejunostomy feeding tube placement during sedation with epidural and local anesthesia versus general anesthesia. Sedation and local anesthesia provided satisfactory conditions for the laparoscopic procedure and less cardiopulmonary depression.[28] Thus, sedation and epidural anesthesia may be considered for critical patients requiring a laparoscopic procedure. Conversion to general anesthesia may be necessary if the duration of the procedure is extended and mechanical ventilation needed to offset increases in $PaCO_2$.

Complications of laparoscopy include hemorrhage, pneumothorax, or puncture of an organ with placement of the veress needle. Splenic enlargement will occur if thiopental is used as the induction agent. Serial packed cell volume (PCV) determination and total protein measurement can help assess the need for blood replacement products. Packed red blood cells and plasma, or whole blood transfusion should be considered if the PCV decreases to less than 20 and the total protein less than 4. Postoperative analgesic needs can be met with parenterally administered opioids. Lidocaine patch application at the port sites can be used to provide regional analgesia without systemic effects.[29]

THORACOSCOPY

When an instrument is placed in the thoracic cavity, the negative pressure of the thorax is compromised. Deliberate collapse of the lung on the operable side is attempted in many instances to improve surgical conditions. One-lung ventilation may be achieved either through selective intubation of one bronchus or the use of a bronchial blocker to improve conditions for endosurgery. Selective intubation can be done blindly or with the aid of an endoscope. Thoracoscopy may also be performed with a more conventional two-lung ventilation technique and the use of smaller tidal volumes to improve surgical conditions. The use of bilateral ventilation techniques decreases general anesthesia time, as selective intubation is not done. Although complete lung collapse does not occur, this tends to be the simplest way to manage the anesthesia for the patient.[30]

One-lung ventilation has minimal cardiopulmonary effects on healthy dogs with an intact chest.[31] Nevertheless, opening the thoracic cavity will have adverse effects on gas exchange and may compromise the patient's oxygenation ability.[32–34] Significant decreases in arterial oxygen partial pressure (PaO_2) and oxygen content can be expected.[32] Significant increases in shunt fraction and physiologic dead space can occur. Arterial partial pressure of carbon dioxide may not be affected.

Whereas laparoscopy requires insufflation of the abdominal cavity, thoracoscopy can be performed with or without carbon dioxide insufflation. Thoracic insufflation decreases cardiac output at low insufflation pressures (3 mmHg) and sustained insufflation should be used with caution.[35]

Monitoring of patients undergoing general anesthesia for thoracoscopy should include capnometry, pulse oximetry, ECG, and blood pressure monitoring. Invasive blood pressure monitoring has the added advantage of arterial catheter placement for easier blood gas analysis. Particular attention should be paid to the patient's ventilation and oxygenation status.

A thoracoscopy procedure in people has the advantage of reduced chest wall trauma, reduced postoperative pain, decreased patient morbidity, and decreased hospitalization time.[36] Thoracoscopy has been used in dogs for the biopsy of pulmonary structures, identification, and ligation of the thoracic duct, pericardectomy, and lung lobectomy, amongst other things.[37–40] However, most of the cardiopulmonary research studies on thoracoscopy have been conducted on healthy dogs. Clinical candidates for thoracoscopy usually have pulmonary compromise, which can hamper their ability to withstand a sustained thoracoscopic procedure. Conversion to thoracotomy may be necessary for patients who desaturate or deteriorate with a lengthy general anesthesia time. One of the most common reasons for conversion to thoracotomy is insufficient lung collapse and visualization of the operative site.[40]

Many of the complications of thoracoscopy are the same as conventional thoracotomy surgery. Decreases in arterial oxygen tension and hypoventilation should be anticipated. The use of 5 cmH$_2$O of positive end expiratory pressure (PEEP) may help with desaturation, especially if one-lung ventilation is used. A mechanical ventilator will help sustain ventilation and free up personnel to monitor the patient. Hemorrhage at the surgical site may occur and the patient should be monitored with serial PCV/total protein measurements. Blood products should be administered if necessary. Plasma or hetastarch can be helpful in maintaining a robust intravascular volume if cardiopulmonary compromise is anticipated.

Animals that experience thoracoscopy may have less pain than patients who experience lateral thoracotomy or median sternotomy, but have analgesic needs that should be addressed nevertheless. Full μ agonist opioids are appropriate analgesic choices for most patients, despite the respiratory depression produced by the drug. Oxygen therapy post procedure may be warranted in many clinical cases.

REFERENCES

1. Richter KP. Laparoscopy in dogs and cats. Vet Clin North Am Small Anim Pract 2001;31:707–27.
2. Seeler DC. Fluid, electrolyte, and blood component therapy. In: Tranquilli WJ, Thurmon JC, Grimm KA, editors. Lumb & Jones' veterinary anesthesia and analgesia. 4th edition. Oxford: Blackwell; 2007. p. 185–201.
3. Holt D, Brockman D. Diagnosis and management of laryngeal disease in the dog and cat. Vet Clin North Am 1994;24:855–71.
4. Jackson AM, Tobias K, Long C, et al. Effects of various anesthetic agents on laryngeal motion during laryngoscopy in normal dogs. Vet Surg 2004;33:102–6.
5. Baker P, Langton JA, Wilson IG, et al. Movements of the vocal cords on induction of anesthesia with thiopentone or propofol. Br J Anesth 1992;69:23–5.
6. Gross ME, Dodam JR, Pope ER, et al. A comparison of thiopental, propofol, and diazepam-ketamine anesthesia for evaluation of laryngeal function in dogs premedicated with butorphanol-glycopyrrolate. J Am Anim Hosp Assoc 2002;38: 503–6.
7. Radlinsky MG, Mason DE, Hodgson D. Transnasal laryngoscopy for the diagnosis of laryngeal paralysis in dogs. J Am Anim Hosp Assoc 2004;40:211–5.
8. Johnson L. Small animal bronchoscopy. Vet Clin North Am Small Anim Pract 2001; 31:691–705.
9. Branson KR. Injectable and alternative anesthetic techniques. In: Tranquilli WJ, Thurmon JC, Grimm KA, editors. Lumb & Jones' veterinary anesthesia and analgesia. 4th edition. Oxford: Blackwell Publishing; 2007. p. 273–99.
10. Tams TR. Gastroscopy. In: Small animal endoscopy. 2nd edition. St Louis (MO): Mosby; 1999. p. 97–172.
11. Zoran DL. Gastroduodenoscopy in the dog and cat. Vet Clin North Am Small Anim Pract 2001;31:631–56.
12. Donaldson LL, Leib MS, Boyd C, et al. Effect of preanesthetic medication on ease of endoscopic intubation of the duodenum in anesthetized dogs. Am J Vet Res 1993;54(9):1489–95.
13. Matz ME, Leib MS, Monroe WE, et al. Evaluation of atropine, glucagon, and metoclopramide for facilitation of endoscopic intubation of the duodenum in dogs. Am J Vet Res 1991;52(12):1948–50.
14. Sap R, Hellebrekers LF. Medetomidine/propofol anaesthesia for gastroduodenal endoscopy in dogs. J Vet Anaesth 1993;20:100–2.
15. Smith AA, Posner LP, Goldstein RE, et al. Evaluation of the effects of premedication on gastroduodenoscopy in cats. J Am Vet Med Assoc 2004;225(4):540–4.
16. Willard MD. Colonoscopy, proctoscopy, and ileoscopy. Vet Clin North Am Small Anim Pract 2001;31:657–69.
17. Leib MS, Baechtel MS, Monroe WE. Complications associated with 355 flexible colonoscopic procedures in dogs. J Vet Intern Med 2004;18:642–6.
18. Marschall H, Bartels F. Life-threatening complications of nasogastric administration of polyethylene glycol-electrolyte solutions (GoLYTELY) for bowel cleansing. Gastrointest Endosc 1998;47:408–10.
19. Noone KE. Rhinoscopy, pharyngoscopy, and laryngoscopy. Vet Clin North Am Small Anim Pract 2001;31:671–89.

20. Quandt JE. Anesthetic considerations for laser, laparoscopy, and thoracoscopic procedures. Clin Tech Small Anim Pract 1999;14:50–5.

21. Don HF, Robson JF. The mechanics of the respiratory system during anesthesia. Anesthesiology 1965;26:168–78.

22. Nunn JF. Effects of anaesthesia on respiration. Br J Anaesth 1990;65:54–62.

23. Gross ME, Jones BD, Bergstresser DR, et al. Effects of abdominal insufflation with nitrous oxide on cardiorespiratory measurements in spontaneously breathing iso-flurane-anesthetized dogs. Am J Vet Res 1993;54(8):1352–8.

24. Bailey JE, Pablo LS. Anesthetic and physiologic considerations for veterinary endosurgery. In: Freeman LJ, editor. Veterinary Endosurgery. St. Louis (MO): Mosby; 1999.

25. Kotrly K, et al. Baroreceptor reflex control of heart rate during isoflurane anesthesia in humans. Anesthesiology 1984;60:173–9.

26. Jois J, et al. Hemodynamic changes during laparoscopic cholecystectomy. Anesth Analg 1993;76:1067–71.

27. Abel F, Pierce J, Guntheroth W. Baroreceptor influence on postural changes in blood pressure and carotid blood flow. Am J Physiol 1963;205:360–4.

28. Hewitt SA, Brisson BA, Sinclair MD, et al. Comparison of cardiopulmonary responses during sedation with epidural and local anesthesia for laparoscopic-assisted jejunostomy feeding tube placement with cardiopulmonary responses during general anesthesia for laparoscopic-assisted or open surgical jejunostomy feeding tube placement in healthy dogs. Am J Vet Res 2007;68(4):358–69.

29. Weil AB, Ko J, Inoue T. The use of lidocaine patches. Compend Contin Educ Vet 2007;29(4):208–16.

30. Gross ME, Dodam JR, Faunt KK. Anesthetic considerations for endoscopy. In: McCarthy T, editor. Veterinary endoscopy for the small animal practitioner. Philadelphia: WB Saunders; 2004. p. 21–9.

31. Cantwell SL, Duke T, Walsh PJ, et al. One-lung versus two-lung ventilation in the closed-chest anesthetized dog: a comparison of cardiopulmonary parameters. Vet Surg 2000;29:365–73.

32. Kudnig ST, Monnet E, Riquelme M, et al. Cardiopulmonary effects of thoracoscopy in anesthetized normal dogs. Vet Anaesth Analg 2004;31:121–8.

33. Faunt KK, Cohn LA, Jones BD. Cardiopulmonary effects of bilateral hemithorax ventilation and diagnostic thoracoscopy in dogs. Am J Vet Res 1998;59:1494–8.

34. Kudnig ST, Monnet E, Riquelme M. Effect of one-lung ventilation on oxygen delivery in anesthetized dogs with an open thoracic cavity. Am J Vet Res 2003; 64:443–8.

35. Daly CM, Swalec-Tobias K, Tobias AH, et al. Cardiopulmonary effects of intrathoracic insufflation in dogs. J Am Anim Hosp Assoc 2002;38:515–20.

36. Lin J, Iannettoni MD. The role of thoracoscopy in the management of lung cancer. Surg Oncol 2003;12:195–200.

37. Swanson SJ, Batirel HF. Video-assisted thoracic surgery (VATS) resection for lung cancer. Surg Clin North Am 2002;82:541–59.

38. Radlinsky MG, Mason DE, Biller DS, et al. Thoracoscopic visualization and ligation of the thoracic duct in dogs. Vet Surg 2002;31:138–46.

39. Dupre GP, Corlouer JP, Bouvy B. Thoracoscopic pericardectomy performed without pulmonary exclusion in 9 dogs. Vet Surg 2001;30:21–7.

40. Lansdowne JL, Monnet E, Twedt DC, et al. Thoracoscopic lung lobectomy for treatment of lung tumors in dogs. Vet Surg 2005;34:530–5.

Diagnostic Rigid Endoscopy: Otoscopy, Rhinoscopy, and Cystoscopy

Clarence A. Rawlings, DVM, PhD

KEYWORDS

- Video otoscopy • Rhinoscopy • Cystoscopy
- Rigid endoscopy

OTOSCOPY
Definition and Tools

Video otoscopy uses video cameras and endoscopic lighting combined with an otoscope to examine the external and middle ear. Video otoscopy is a vast improvement over traditional otoscopy because the image is magnified and projected on a monitor compared with visualizing through a small otoscope loop (**Fig. 1**). Flushing with fluids during anesthesia concurrently clears the field of view. Veterinarians can markedly improve their examination of the ear and, equally important, the client can gain an appreciation of the disease process. Practitioners using video otoscopy strongly vouch for the subsequent improvement in client compliance and patient's ear care.

Instrumentation for video otoscopy requires the standard camera, light, image processor, and digital capture system in a standard endoscopy tower (Karl Storz Veterinary Enoscopy, Goleta, California). The camera and light cable are connected to a video otoscopy cone and small diameter endoscopes (**Fig. 2**). Only the video otoscope cone is required for awake and sedated examinations in the outpatient arena. Air is the optical medium in wakeful patients.

Smaller endoscopes and otoscopy cones can be used while infusing fluid in anesthetized patients. Smaller diameters used include 1.9-mm and 2.7-mm endoscopes encased in cystoscope sheaths. These endoscopes have a 30° viewing angle, and the sheaths have an operating channel. Arthroscope sheaths also work well and provide an excellent avenue for irrigation; however, they do not have an instrument channel. Ancillary equipment includes flushing catheters, biopsy forceps, foreign body removal forceps, curettes, ear loops, mosquito forceps, alligator forceps, and suction.

Department of Small Animal Medicine and Surgery, College of Veterinary Medicine, University of Georgia, Athens, GA 30602-7390, USA
E-mail address: c_rawlings@bellsouth.net

Vet Clin Small Anim 39 (2009) 849–868
doi:10.1016/j.cvsm.2009.05.010
0195-5616/09/$ – see front matter © 2009 Published by Elsevier Inc.

vetsmall.theclinics.com

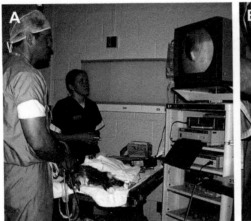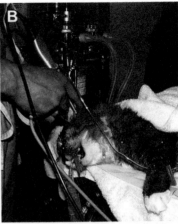

Fig. 1. (*A, B*) Video otoscopy used to examine a cat's ear during anesthesia. Examination is carried out before and after thorough cleaning. Note that the operator is looking at the monitor, which is opposite the ear from the operator. Swabs for cytology and culture, if indicated, are done before cleaning. A deep culture should be obtained if the tympanic membrane is ruptured or if there is obvious otitis media. A short movie of the ear mites seen in this cat can be downloaded from the website, www.vet.uga.edu/mis.

Indications and Case Selection

Ear diseases are extremely common problems in general veterinary practice.[1,2] Dermatologists use the ear as a sentinel for generalized skin diseases, for example, dietary-based allergic dermatitis. Acute signs of otitis externa include pinnal and otic hyperemia, edema, and excoriation (**Fig. 3**). Chronicity leads to hyperplasia and mineralization of the ear canal. Most patients have an abundance of malodorous discharge and pruritus, as evidenced by head shaking and pain. A thorough dermatologic examination is essential, and the ear should be cleaned as the first step in treatment. Most dogs and cats have otitis externa, but otitis media must be ruled out for

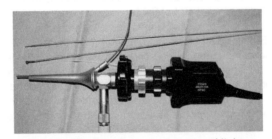

Fig. 2. An otoscopy cone used with an endoscopic camera and light source. Either a suction irrigation machine (Vet Pump 2) with a 5 Fr red rubber urinary catheter or a "Y" shaped stopcock attachment with integrated operating channel can be connected to the infusion channel. During anesthesia, video otoscopy is commonly done with a rigid endoscope, such as a 2.7-mm diameter, 18-cm long scope with either an arthroscopy or cystoscopy sheath (Karl Storz Veterinary Enoscopy, Goleta, California). The cystoscope has an inflow and efflux port in addition to an operating channel, whereas the arthroscope sheath is smaller and only has an inflow port. The cystoscope has a rounded, more benign tip than the arthroscope. Smaller rigid scopes can also be used for the ear.

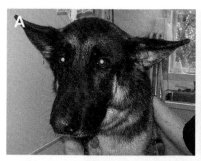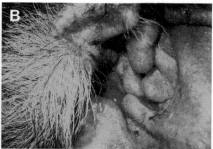

Fig. 3. This 5-year-old German shepherd has a history of skin disease. Both ears had a 4-month history of mucopurulent discharge and pain, as reflected by his ear carriage (*A*). The ears had previously transiently improved with cleaning and prednisolone. The ears are severely inflamed and erythematous, typical of an allergic response (*B*).

effective topical treatment. Neurologic and otoscopic examinations are helpful in diagnosing otitis media. Indications for video otoscopy are (1) clinical signs of ear disease, (2) otic odor, discharge, or pain, (3) older dogs presenting for geriatric examination, (4) breeds commonly affected by ear disease, and (5) chronic skin disease.[1,2] Video otoscopy done in the outpatient room is a cursory examination at best and should be restricted to evaluation of a healthy ear with no clinical signs or to identification of problems requiring more intensive examination. When the ear is inflamed, painful, or filled with purulent material, anesthesia is required to perform a thorough cleaning and examination. The combination of anesthesia, improved video images, and irrigation through the scope improves visualization of the ear canal and tympanic membrane, and it is ideal for diagnosing otitis media. Skull radiographs are helpful, but limited in their diagnostic sensitivity for middle ear disease. Computed tomography (CT) and magnetic resonance imagining (MRI) are useful for examining the tympanic bulla but are expensive compared with video otoscopy. Undiagnosed and incompletely managed middle ear disease is a common cause of persistent otitis externa. In addition, failure to rid the ear of exudate makes it nearly impossible to appropriately medicate the external ear.

Typical Abnormalities

The most frequent abnormalities are an abundance of malodorous discharge and inflammation. An ear swab for cystologic examination for yeast and bacteria should be taken before ear cleaning, and cultures are easily obtained. The ear canal may be narrow as a result of congenital or acquired disease and may be obstructed by hyperplasia. Other findings include ear mites, mass lesions, and foreign bodies. Masses should be sampled for histologic examination. Multiple causes of ear diseases include infection (bacteria, yeast, or fungal), foreign bodies (foxtails, plant material, and exudate), allergy (atopy, food, or contact), endocrinopathies (hypothyroidism or sex hormone imbalance), seborrhea (primary or secondary), conformation (stenotic, hypertrichosis), immune-mediated diseases (pemphigus or lupus), benign masses (polyps or hyperplasia), and neoplasia (ceruminous gland adenocarcinoma, squamous cell carcinoma). Representative cases of the above lesions are presented in **Figs. 4–9**.

Patient Management After Endoscopy

In the first few hours, postoperative pain is managed by mild oral analgesics, such as tramadol, which is often dispensed at discharge. Many patients require

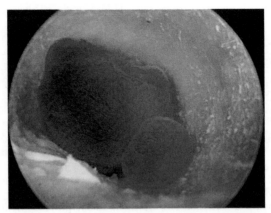

Fig. 4. Video-otoscopic image of the left ear of a 5-year-old neutered male cat. The left ear had had a bloody discharge, first observed 1 year previously. Biopsy was an inflammatory polyp. Treatment requires removal of the polyp from both the bulla and eutaschian tube. This is done either by ventral bulla osteotomy or by otoscopy, in which the septum between the cranial lateral and larger ventral medial tympanic bulla compartment is perforated sufficient to debride the medial compartment.

corticosteroids as a part of their treatment, or nonsteroid analgesic drugs can be used.[3] Indications for surgery are persistent otitis that fails to respond or does not appear to be likely to recover with medical treatment. Otitis externa and otitis media require persistent medical management by the veterinarian and client. Once ear disease recurs, the ear must be regularly examined by video otoscopy. It aids in managing middle ear disease by lavage and cleansing of the middle ear through the ruptured tympanic membrane. Failure to maintain an acceptable external canal lumen is an indication for ear surgery. Having worked in a variety of practices as a referral general surgeon, the author has observed that the effectiveness of medical treatment has markedly altered the number of patients operated. Aggressive and persistent

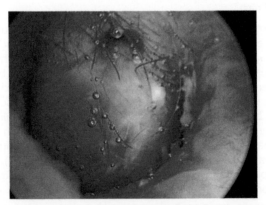

Fig. 5. Video-otoscopic view of the left ear of a 4-year-old female spayed mixed dog with recurrent left side otitis externa. The biopsy diagnosis was a benign papilloma with moderate monocytic to neutrophilic perivascular dermatitis. This mass should be surgically resected with selection of the surgical procedure based on mass location and size. Resection may be local or as extensive as total ear canal ablation.

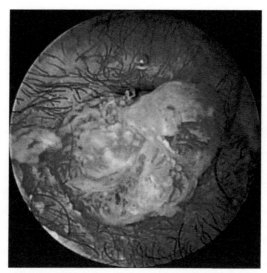

Fig. 6. Video-otoscopic view of the left ear of a 10-year-old male cocker spaniel. The histologic diagnosis was a well-differentiated ceruminous adenocarcinoma. A fine-needle aspirate from the mandibular lymph node was negative for cancer cells. Treatment was believed to be successful after total ear-canal ablation with a lateral bulla osteotomy, when the surgical margins were negative for cancer.

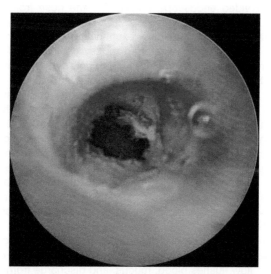

Fig. 7. Video-otoscopic view in a 7-year-old male Brittany spaniel with a 1-year history of otitis externa and media, including a head tilt. This ear had previously had a ventral bulla osteotomy and lateral ear resection. Video otoscopy during sedation on the previous day had found a bulging tympanic membrane with dark material in the middle ear. At this time, the tympanic membrane was ruptured. If long-time ear management is persistent, this ear can be managed by aggressive flushing using the otoscope to insure thorough cleaning.

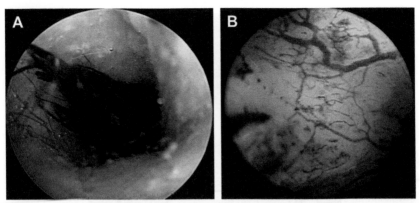

Fig. 8. Video-otoscopic image of a 1-year-old spayed female miniature poodle with recurrent bilateral ear infections. (*A*) Weed awns were present in the external ear canal with penetration through the tympanic membrane into the middle ear. Tissue and debris within the middle ear were removed using the video otoscope. (*B*) The clean inside of the bulla is seen after debridement. The bulla is so thoroughly cleaned that individual red blood cells can be seen within vessels in this image and in movie recordings.

video otoscpic treatment can markedly reduce the requirement for end-stage ear surgery.

RHINOSCOPY
Definition and Tools

Rhinoscopy uses a video endoscope to examine the nose from the naris to the pharynx. The most useful endoscope is the 2.7-mm diameter, 18-cm long endoscope with a 3.5-mm outer diameter arthroscopy examination sheath (Karl Storz Veterinary Enoscopy, Goleta, California). The preferred biopsy device is a 3-mm oval biopsy forceps, which procures large samples for imprint cytology and formalin-fixed pathology (**Fig. 10**). This combination of endoscope and biopsy forceps requires some practice, as they are passed parallel to each other during sampling; the tips of the forceps may not always remain in sight when learning the technique. Other rhinoscopic tools include a 2.7-mm endoscope with a 14.5-mm (4 × 5.5 mm) cystoscope with a biopsy channel for flexible biopsy forceps, a 1.9-mm endoscope with a 10 Fr cystoscope, and smaller diameter arthroscopes. Cats and small dogs are examined with the 1.9-mm cystoscope or an arthroscope. The cystoscopes have a biopsy channel, which is seldom used for sampling because of the small sample size collected with this method. Routine examination of the nasal pharynx is possible with a rigid endoscope, decreasing the need for retroflex endoscopy of the nasal pharynx through the oral cavity.[4]

High fluid flow with a balanced electrolyte solution during rhinoscopy reduces the effect of iatrogenic hemorrhage on imaging and provides some distention of the optical space. High flow flushes blood, mucus, and discharge from the field of view; this and the 30° viewing angle are two benefits of rigid, rather than a flexible, endoscopy. Fluid drainage can be improved by ensuring that there is no pharyngeal obstruction to flow and by placing the nose over the end of the examination table, providing effluent drainage into a trash can. The search for abnormalities should be anatomically systematic and initially directed toward the anticipated problem, based on clinical signs and imaging tests. Both nasal passages are explored before biopsy. Samples

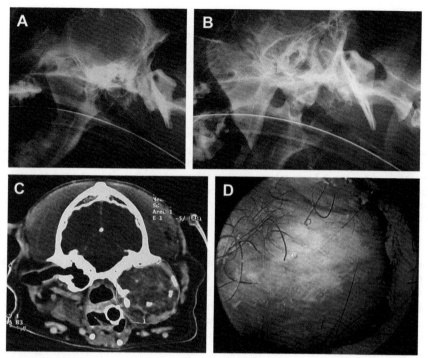

Fig. 9. Skull radiographs from an 11-year-old neutered male dog with left otitis and head tilt. The dog was reluctant to open his mouth. A previous biopsy was interpreted as being a ceruminous adenoma, but the referring veterinarian suspected a more aggressive lesion. The right bulla (A) seems to be normal in contrast to the left bulla (B), which has evidence of lysis and new bone formation. (C) A contrast CT identified a left ear mass that is vascular, has osteolysis, has new bone formation, and is expansive enough to involve the temporal mandibular joint. (D) Video-otoscopic image of the mass as viewed from the ear canal. The mass appeared to be mural, but the surface did not have a proliferative character. A biopsy core needle from the mass was diagnosed as a ceruminous adenocarcinoma. The behavior of spreading and histology was worse than the previous diagnosis of ceruminous adenoma.

of the most obvious lesions should be taken first, and multiple biopsies should be obtained, preferably with the 3-mm biopsy or larger forceps. Although hemorrhage can complicate any rhinoscopy, bleeding is more controllable with the high fluid infusion rates by using the 2.7-mm rigid endoscope with an examination sheath. Significant hemorrhage has not been problematic after rhinoscopy, even with extensive curettage of nasal cancer.

Indications and Case Selection

Signs representing indications for rhinoscopy include persistent nasal discharge, epistaxis, sneezing, stertor, choking, nasal pruritus typical of a foreign body, nasal pain or increased sensitivity, facial swelling, or history of foreign body inhalation.[4] Diagnostic tests include history, physical examination, complete blood count, chemistry profile, and coagulation profile. Contrast CT has replaced traditional radiography in many practices. Advanced imaging (CT and MRI) is superior to radiographs for determining the site and extent of nasal disease. Foreign bodies and cancer can be

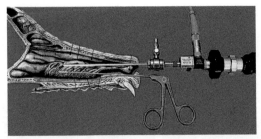

Fig.10. A 2.7-mm arthroscope with 3-mm biopsy cup forceps used for rhinoscopy (Karl Storz Veterinary Enoscopy, Goleta, California). The arthroscope has the highest flow of the sheaths used for the 2.7-mm telescope, thus vigorously flushing hemorrhage and debris from the nose. The 3-mm biopsy cup forceps provides a large, diagnostic sample, although the combined use of the scope and biopsy cup forceps requires practice. Diagnostic samples may be obtained from the vigorous nasal flushing.

specifically identified and localized. The anatomic knowledge gained speeds up and simplifies the endoscopic examination.

A wide variety of anesthetic agents can be used, but maintaining a deep plane of anesthesia is essential for rhinoscopy, as the nasal cavity is very sensitive, and inadequate anesthesia can produce pain, movement, and sneezing. In addition to analgesic drugs, an infraorbital local nerve block may be performed (**Fig. 11**A, B). The trachea must be protected with a properly inflated endotracheal cuff during rhinoscopy and fluid infusion.

Typical Abnormalities

Neoplasia (see **Fig. 11; Fig. 12**) is a common cause of clinical signs and nasal airway obstruction, and rarely will obstruction be associated with stricture, such as a choanal stricture (**Fig. 13**). Nonobstructive diseases include neoplasia, allergic inflammation (rhinitis), fungal infection, foreign bodies (**Fig. 14**), and parasites. Multiple biopsies are taken in every case, and imprint cytology and cultures may also be obtained. A complete examination must also include the oral cavity and upper airway and fine-needle aspirates of the mandibular lymph nodes when neoplasia is suspected. Representative lesions are presented in **Figs. 11–14**.

Patients with nasal cancer may undergo transnares curettage at the time of diagnostic rhinoscopy. Surgical resection of nasal tumors may prolong survival time and improve quality of life for cancer patients.[5] Debulking provides large, diagnostic samples for histopathologic examination (see **Fig. 11**E). Patients quickly overcome clinical signs of nasal obstruction, and repeated curettage can prolong survival and improve quality of life.

Patient Management After Endoscopy

Keeping the nose directed downward during recovery encourages drainage after rhinoscopy. Postoperative analgesics and sedatives are used to reduce the pain, stress, and sneezing. Patients should be maintained in a recovery ward and analgesic drugs should be given before perceived pain. Some clinicians discharge patients the evening after rhinoscopy if the patient has completely recovered from anesthesia. The author prefers to monitor patients for the first night after rhinoscopy.

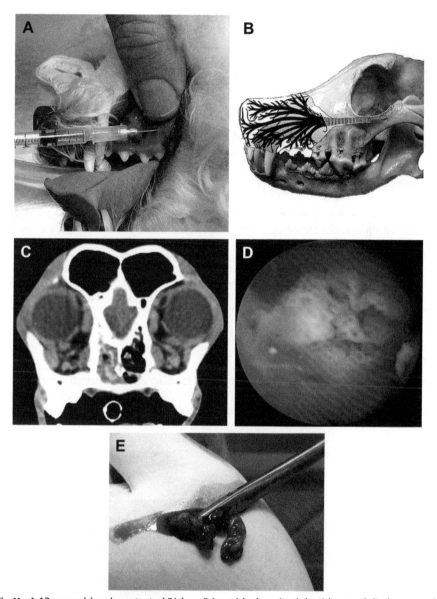

Fig. 11. A 12-year-old male castrated Bichon Frise with chronic, right side, nasal discharge and sneezing. Before rhinoscopy, an infraorbital nerve block is performed by local anesthetic injection at the infraorbital foramen (*A*). The foramen can be palpated as being dorsal and just cranial to the fourth premolar tooth (*B*). The caudal area of the right nasal canal is obstructed with tissue as viewed by CT (*C*), and this mass can be seen on rhinoscopy (*D*). In addition to the initial biopsy, this mass was treated by curettage, and some of this sample is seen (*E*). After curettage, the nasal cavity was vigorously flushed. The histologic diagnosis was a solid and acinar adenocarcinoma. Radiation treatment and reexamination by rhinoscopy were recommended.

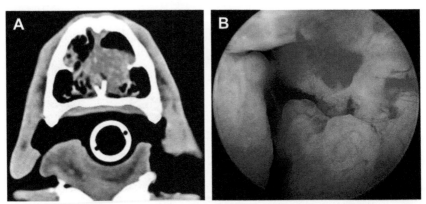

Fig. 12. This 16-year-old spayed female German shepherd mix had a history of left-side epistaxis with a previous rhinoscopic diagnosis of cancer. The owner declined the recommendation for radiation therapy. The mass, which had crossed the midline (*A*), was identified from contrast CT. The rhinoscopic image of the mass showed it to be proliferative (*B*) and the histologic diagnosis was an undifferentiated sarcoma of the nasal submucosa. This tumor was removed by curettage at the time of rhinoscopy and again 5 months later. Improved breathing developed soon after rhinoscopic curettage, and survival was for 2 years.

CYSTOSCOPY
Definition and Tools

Traditional cystoscopy, in practice, may be used for diagnosis, for calculi removal, and for repair of ectopic ureters. Compared with a traditional cystotomy, the magnified images are more revealing, as cystoscopy distends the urogenital system with fluid and does not require a hemorrhage-producing incision.[6–8] After diagnostic procedures such as survey radiographs and ultrasonography, cystoscopy is more efficient, increases diagnostic accuracy, provides the ability to selectively obtain biopsies, and

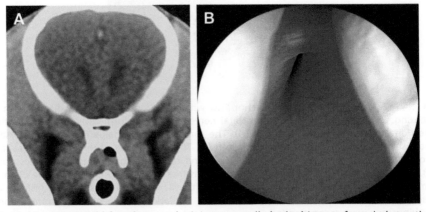

Fig. 13. This 10-year-old female spayed miniature poodle had a history of nasal obstruction and open mouth breathing. The stricture is seen on the contrast CT (*A*) and during rhinoscopy (*B*). Rhinoscopic resection was done using radiofrequency placed through the operating channel of a cystoscope.

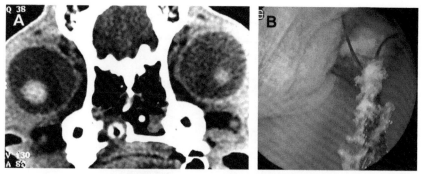

Fig. 14. A 2-year-old male neutered pug had a 3-month history of snorting, coughing, licking, and serous nasal discharge. A foreign body and lysis of the hard palate are seen on the contrast CT (*A*). The mass was a kernel of unpopped popcorn, which was removed with a three-wire basket catheter (*B*).

is easier to apply in clinical practice than contrast procedures and CT.[7] Cystoscopy has become the treatment tool for ectopic ureters, calculi removal, lithotripsy, polypectomy, and transitional cell carcinoma.[9–13]

Transurethral cystoscopy in the female dog and cat is performed with a rigid cystoscope. Cystoscopes with a 30° angle provide some degree of side viewing and direct advancement of the endoscope cranially within the urogenital tract. The most frequently used endoscope is a 2.7-mm diameter, 18-cm long cystoscope with a 14.5 Fr sheath (**Fig. 15**), which can be used in female dogs as small as 5 kg. In dogs larger than 15 to 20 kg, the 2.7-mm cystoscope can usually be used to examine the urethral and bladder outflow, but it is too short to do a thorough bladder examination or treatment. In these larger female dogs, a 3.5- or 4-mm diameter, 30-cm long cystoscope is preferred. In female dogs smaller than 5 kg and female cats, a 1.9-mm diameter, 18-cm long cystoscope is required.[6] The angled viewing increases the examination capabilities, as the endoscope can be rotated 360°. Infusion of a balanced electrolyte solution permits flushing and distention of the optical space.

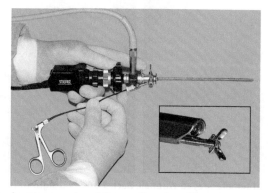

Fig. 15. The standard cystoscope is a 2.7-mm diameter, 18-cm long scope placed in a 14.5 Fr cystoscope sheath. The sheath has a port for fluid infusion and outflow, and an operating channel (Karl Storz Veterinary Enoscopy, Goleta, California). A variety of instruments from diagnostic biopsy cup forceps to treatment instruments can be passed through the operating channel.

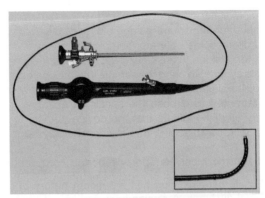

Fig. 16. The urethra of male dogs is examined with a flexible 2.5- to 2.8-mm urethroscope using the endoscopic camera and light sources. This scope can be passed from the penile orifice or from the bladder during a laparoscopic-assisted cystoscopy. It is an excellent technique for identifying calculi and lesions in the male urethra. The same light and camera systems are used for this flexible fiberoptic scope as with the 2.7-mm rigid cystoscope shown here.

Transurethral cystoscopy of male dogs is done with a flexible urethroscope (**Fig. 16**). It is possible to examine the urinary system with a 1.9-mm rigid cystoscope after perineal urethrostomy in the cat. Most small animal patients can also be examined with laparoscopic-assisted cystoscopy.

Indications and Case Selection

Indications for cystoscopy include chronic or recurrent urinary tract infection, hematuria, dysuria, stranguria, pollakuria, trauma, calculi, incontinence, abnormal urine sediment, and follow-up results of abdominal radiographs and ultrasound. If a problem

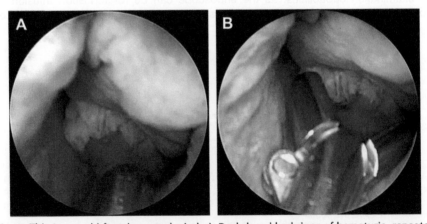

Fig. 17. This 1-year-old female spayed wirehair Dachshund had signs of hematuria, repeated attempts to urinate, urinary tract infection, and cystic calculi. (*A*) During cystoscopy to remove the calculi, the mass could be seen slightly projecting into the vestibule from the urethral meatus and then continuing cranially in the urethra. (*B*) Three-millimeter oval biopsy forceps were used to obtain a sample of the protruding mass, which was diagnosed as a transitional cell carcinoma.

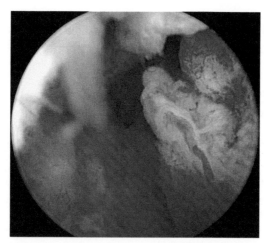

Fig. 18. This 9-year-old female spayed dog had a 4-month history of inappropriate urination, intermittent hematuria, and stranguria. The dog also had diabetes mellitus. Proliferative masses were seen throughout the length of the urethra, and this mass was reduced in size using a diode laser through the operating channel. In addition, the inguinal lymph node was aspirated and found to be metastasis of transition cell carcinoma from the urethra.)

is difficult to diagnose or resolve, cytoscopy is a quick and direct approach to diagnosis.[6] Cystoscopy should be considered an essential part of the database for diagnosing most urinary problems. Other diagnostic tools include history, physical examination, complete blood count, serum chemistry profile, and urinalysis. Urine is best obtained by cystocentesis, with a portion of the sample submitted for culture and susceptibility testing. In addition to using cytoscopy for diagnosis, the operating channel allows passage of grasping forceps, basket catheters, and energy devices for treatment (see **Fig. 15**). The main disadvantage of cystoscopy is the need for general

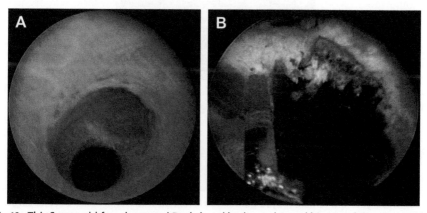

Fig. 19. This 6-year-old female spayed Dachshund had a prolonged history of dysuria, and for several years, starting after her spay, she would yelp when placed in lateral recumbency. A stricture was present in the cranial area of the urethra (*A*). The stricture was resected using a diode laser passed through the operating channel (*B*).

anesthesia; however, the procedure is typically quick and minimally invasive. Other risks of cystoscopy include urethral or bladder trauma or perforation and bladder overdistention.

Typical Abnormalities

Cystoscopy should be performed in a consistent anatomic manner, despite the tendency to focus on abnormal findings. The vestibule should be examined before proceeding into the urethra or vagina.[7] Urinary tract inflammation is commonly small inflammatory foci, especially in cases of infection. Typical findings in the urethra are inflammatory foci, calculi, ectopic ureters, and tumors, most commonly transitional cell carcinoma.[14,15] Other causes of dysuria include prostatic abscess or cysts, granulomatous masses, strictures, trauma, and urethral contraction caused by bladder-urethral sphincter reflex dyssynergia.[7] Other masses obstructing flow include inflammatory polyps and blood clots. Straining can be produced by vaginal

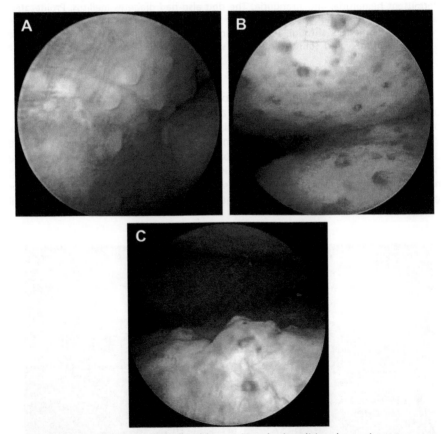

Fig. 20. This 7-year-old female spayed golden retriever had traditional ectopic ureter surgery performed at 6 months of age, but had had recurrent incontinence and urinary tract infections. At the time of this examination, urinary tract infection and a recessed vulva with overhanging perivulvar skin were present. Inflammatory foci were present in the vestibule (*A*), urethra (*B*), and bladder (*C*).

and vestibular masses. Other lesions include idiopathic renal hematuria[16] and extra-luminal masses.

Older dogs with incontinence and recurrent urinary tract infections may not have apparent anatomic abnormalities, but the elimination of potential causes is helpful for case management. Many dogs with recurrent urinary tract infection have predisposing factors, such as a juvenile vulva with excessive skin folds, calculi, foreign bodies, or masses. Calculi in females can be diagnosed by rigid cystoscopy and in male dogs using flexible urethroscopy. Calculi may be removed by transurethral cystoscopy in female dogs when the calculi are only two to three times the diameter of the largest cystoscope appropriate for the patient. Passing 3- to 4-wire basket catheters with a flexible urethroscope through the cystoscope's operating channel for stone removal may be possible in male dogs. Calculi in male cats may be removed by transurethral cystoscopy when a perineal urethrostomy has also been performed. Cystic calculi and most urethral calculi can be removed by a laparoscopic-assisted cystoscopy in both male and female dogs and cats.[17] Endoscopic surgical treatment can also be done for strictures, intraluminal masses, intraluminal foreign bodies, and transitional cell carcinoma. Representative lesions are presented in **Figs. 17–25**.

Calculi too large for removal by transurethral cystoscopy in female dogs and cats and calculi in male dogs and cats can be removed using cystoscopy, done as a laparoscopic-assisted procedure (**Fig. 26**).[11] Two laparoscopic trocars are used for laparoscopic-assisted cystoscopy. The cranial portion of the bladder is lifted to the abdominal wall and a minicystotomy is performed. A 2.7-mm cystoscope is placed

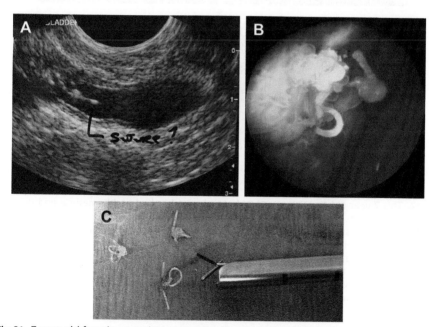

Fig. 21. 7-year-old female spayed West Highland terrier had recurrent urinary tract infections for several years. A cystotomy to remove calculi had been performed 7 weeks previously, and the dog now has hematuria and frequent straining in attempts to urinate. There were also bilateral nephroliths. Suture was suspected on ultrasound (A), found on cystoscopy (B), and removed (C). At the time of cystoscopy, urine cultures were negative. Monitoring for infection must be continued, and further management of nephroliths should be considered.

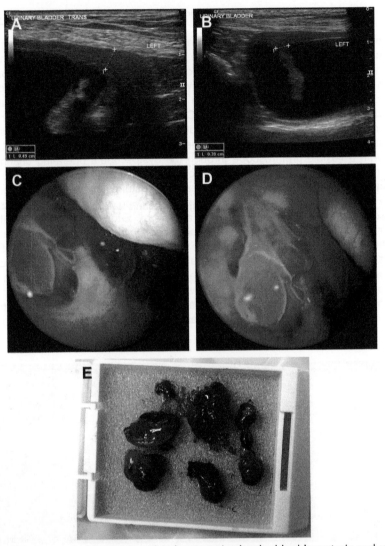

Fig. 22. This 7-year-old female spayed Doberman pinscher had had hematuria and urinary incontinence for at least 2 years. The owner thought that the signs were seasonal, being more severe in the summers. Urinary tract infections were common, and there was a recessed vulva. Although episioplasty was recommended, the owner only gave consent for noninvasive treatment. The ultrasound examination (*A* and *B*) found three masses attached to the bladder wall, with the primary ruleout being inflammatory polyps. The three polyps were found during cystoscopy (*C* and *D*) and removed by diode laser and snares (*E*). Histology confirmed inflammatory polyps.

into the bladder for examination and removal of calculi. For cats and small dogs, a 1.9-mm cystoscope is used. The urethra of female dogs can be examined with the rigid cystoscope and a 2.5- to 2.8-mm fiberoptic scope is attached to the camera for examination of the urethra in male dogs. Urethral strictures proximal to the os penis from previous obstruction and trauma may be identified, and knowledge of such strictures

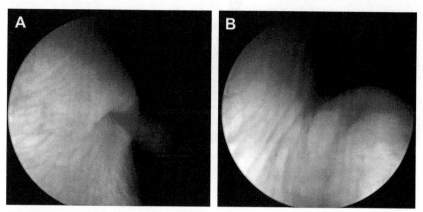

Fig. 23. This 4-year-old female spayed mixed-breed dog had a 2-month history of hematuria and stranguria. Response to antibiotics and corticosteroids had been transient. Ultrasound and an excretory urogram were unremarkable. Cystoscopy found hemorrhage in the urine exiting the right ureter (A), but not the left (B).

can justify a scrotal urethrostomy. Advantages of this technique are limited peritoneal contamination with urine, improved visibility, examination of the entire lower urinary tract, and more complete removal of calculi. Cystic polyps can also be removed by laparoscopic-assisted cystoscopy,[18] or some can be resected by transurethral cystoscopy.

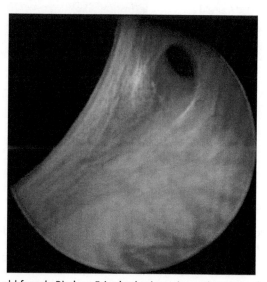

Fig. 24. This 2-year-old female Bischon Frise had urinary incontinence and urinary tract infection. A mildly dilated ectopic ureter was seen on the left side. Diode laser resection of the tissue between the urethra and the left side intramural ectopic ureter resolved the incontinence.

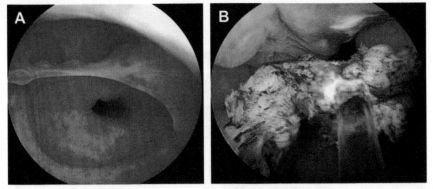

Fig. 25. This 2-year-old female Siberian husky had urinary incontinence. Bilateral ectopic ureter was present; the right ureter was very dilated (*A*). The diode laser was used to resect the membrane between the right intramural ectopic ureter and the urethra (*B*).

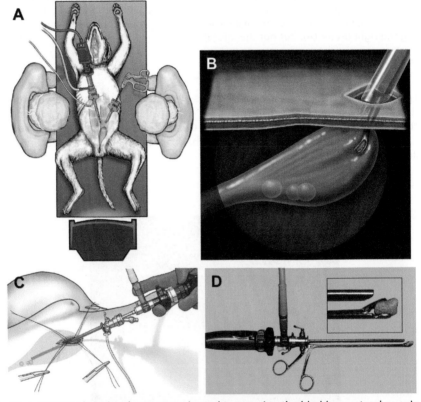

Fig. 26. Laparoscopic-assisted cystoscopy is used to examine the bladder, ureteral openings, and urethra, and to remove the calculi that cannot be removed by transurethral cystoscopy. Laparoscopy (*A*) is done to identify and lift the cranial portion of the bladder to the abdominal wall (*B*). The caudal trocar site is enlarged enough to permit securing the bladder to the abdominal wall and to perform a minicystotomy for placing the cystoscope into the bladder lumen (*C*). Calculi are removed by using either wire-basket catheters through the operating channel or a variety of grasping devices passed parallel to the cystoscope (*D*). After the calculi are removed, small calculi can be flushed and aspirated from the bladder. The urethra should be examined using either the rigid cystoscope in a female dog or a flexible fiberoptic scope in the male dog.

Patient Management After Cystoscopy

Mild analgesic narcotic drugs are routinely provided after transurethral cystoscopy. If additional surgery, such as resection of urethral neoplasia or episoplasty, has been performed, longer acting and more potent narcotics are used. Nonsteroidal drugs or tramadol can be dispensed with the patient. Pain management after laparoscopic-assisted cystoscopy is managed in similar fashion to any laparoscopy procedure.

Control of preexisting urinary infection should be attempted before surgery. If infection persists, culture of bladder mucosa should be considered. Regardless of control of urinary infection, the potential contamination dictates the use of perioperative antibiotics. After cystoscopy, urinary tract infection should be treated with antibiotics, based on susceptibility testing of either urine or bladder mucosal culture. After completion of antibiotic administration, a centesis-obtained urinalysis and culture should be repeated approximately five to seven days later to ensure elimination of the infection.

Incontinent patients are candidates for phenylpropanolamine (1.5 mg/kg given 3 times a day) or estrogen treatment. Persistent incontinence in the face of negative culture and cystoscopy may be treated by colposuspension or cystoscopic-guided urtheral injection augmentation.[19]

SUMMARY

Endoscopy for video otoscopy, rhinoscopy, and cystoscopy is useful for high-quality practices and should be the standard of practice for the complete specialty hospital. These are quick and highly accurate diagnostic procedures. Recent developments have also provided many endoscopic treatments, most of which can be incorporated into general practice and specialty hospitals. Expertise can be developed by many veterinarians, but requires working closely with an experienced endoscopist or participating in "hands-on" introductory endoscopy courses teaching rigid video otoscopy, rhinoscopy, and cystoscopy. The equipment cost and learning curve are more favorable than many other new practice technologies. Clients are receptive to the value of endoscopy; the images and movies are excellent aids for client education and monitoring of disease progression or regression.

REFERENCES

1. Angus JC, Campbell KL. Uses and indications for video-otoscopy in small animal practice. Vet Clin North Am Small Anim Pract 2001;31:809–28.
2. Cole LK. Otoscopic evaluation of the ear canal. Vet Clin North Am Small Anim Pract 2004;34:397–410.
3. Palmeiro BS, Morris DO, Wiemelt SP, et al. Evaluation of outcome of otitis media after lavage of the typmpanic bulla and long-term antimicrobial drug treatment in dogs: 44 cases (1998–2002). J Am Vet Med Assoc 2004;225:548.
4. McCarthy TC. Rhinoscopy: the diagnostic approach to chronic nasal disease. In: McCarthy TC, editor. Veterinary endoscopy for the small animal practitioner. St Louis: Elsevier Saunders; 2005. p. 137–200.
5. Adams WM, Bjorling DE, McAnulty JE, et al. Outcome of accelerated radiotherapy alone or accelerated radiotherapy followed by exenteration of the nasal cavity in dogs with intranasal neoplasia: 53 cases (1990–2002). J Am Vet Med Assoc 2005;227(6):936–41.

6. Cannizzo KL, McLoughlin MA, Chew DJ. Uroendoscopy, evaluation of the lower urinary tract. Vet Clin North Am Small Pract 2001;31:789–807.

7. McCarthy TC. Cystoscopy. In: McCarthy TC, editor. Veterinary endoscopy for the small animal practitioner. St Louis: Elsevier Saunders; 2005:49–135.

8. Senior DF. Cystoscopy. In: Tams TR, editor. Small animal endoscopy. 2nd edition. St Louis: Mosby; 1999.

9. McCarthy TC. Transurethral cystoscopy and diode laser incision to correct an ectopic ureter. Vet Medicine 2006;101(9):558–9.

10. Adams L, Berent A, Moore A, et al. Laser lithotripsy for the removal of uroliths in 73 dogs. J Am Vet Med Assoc 2008;232(7):1026–34.

11. Defarges A, Dunn M. Use of electrohydraulic lithotripsy in 28 dogs with bladder and urethral calculi. J Vet Intern Med 2008;22(6):1267–73.

12. Bevan JM, Lulich, et al. Comparison of laser lithotripsy and cystotomy for the management of dogs with urolithiasis. JAVMA 2009;234:1286–94.

13. Lulich JP, Osborne CA, et al. Efficacy and safety of laser lithotripsy in fragmentation of urocystoliths and urethroliths for removal in dogs. JAVMA 2009;234:1279–85.

14. Phillips BS. Bladder tumors in dogs and cats. Compend Cont Educ Pract Vet 1999;21:540–64.

15. Valli VE, Norris A, Jacobs RM, et al. Pathology of canine bladder and urethral cancer and correlation with tumor progression and survival. J Comp Pathol 1995;113:113–30.

16. Kaufman AC, Barsanti JA, Selcer BA. Benign essential hematuria in dogs. Compend Cont Educ Pract Vet 1994;16:1317.

17. Rawlings CA, Barsanti JA, Mahaffey MB, et al. Use of laparoscopic-assisted cystoscopy for removal of calculi in dogs. J Am Vet Med Assoc 2003;222:759–61.

18. Rawlings CA. Resection of inflammatory polyps in dogs using laparoscopic-assisted cystoscopy. J Am Anim Hosp Assoc 2007;43:1–5.

19. Rawlings CA, Barsanti JA, Mahaffey MB, et al. Evaluation of colposuspension for treatment of incontinence in spayed female dogs. J Am Vet Med Assoc 2001;219:770–5.

Airway Evaluation and Flexible Endoscopic Procedures in Dogs and Cats: Laryngoscopy, Transtracheal Wash, Tracheobronchoscopy, and Bronchoalveolar Lavage

Kate E. Creevy, DVM, MS

KEYWORDS

• Bronchoscopy • Respiratory tract • Airway cytology
• Canine • Feline

Flexible endoscopy is routinely used to visualize and sample the upper and lower respiratory tract. Laryngoscopy is indicated for evaluation of the structure and function of the larynx. Tracheal washes include transtracheal and endotracheal techniques and are minimally invasive diagnostic procedures that blindly collect samples from the respiratory tract. Both of these procedures can be performed in minutes, with limited need for special equipment. For this reason, a wash may be performed as a screening test, before more invasive airway diagnostics. Tracheobronchoscopy is a more invasive diagnostic procedure that allows direct visualization of the lumen and mucosa of the respiratory tree and also facilitates sampling by means of bronchial brushing, biopsy, and bronchoalveolar lavage (BAL). In cases of foreign bodies or aspirated material, tracheobronchoscopy may become a therapeutic intervention. These procedures are reviewed and compared in this report.

LARYNGOSCOPY

Laryngoscopy is indicated for dogs or cats with voice change, stridor, increased inspiratory effort, or exercise intolerance as a primary respiratory sign.[1–3] Most clinicians

Department of Small Animal Medicine and Surgery, College of Veterinary Medicine, University of Georgia, 501 DW Brooks Drive, Athens, GA 30602, USA
E-mail address: creevy@uga.edu

Vet Clin Small Anim 39 (2009) 869–880
doi:10.1016/j.cvsm.2009.05.001
0195-5616/09/$ – see front matter © 2009 Elsevier Inc. All rights reserved.

perform this procedure from an oral approach under sedation, with an intubating laryngoscope or penlight and tongue depressor; however, use of a flexible endoscope for laryngoscopy from an oral or transnasal approach (in dogs greater than 20 kg) is also reported.[4] The use of flexible endoscopy from an oral approach enables closer inspection of the area and facilitates taking photographs, if needed, whereas the transnasal approach may decrease the need for deep sedation.[3,4]

In each of these approaches, dogs and cats require sedation. The ideal protocol for this purpose is controversial, because of the concern of interfering with laryngeal function. When using an oral approach, whether by means of an intubating laryngoscope or a flexible endoscope, a depth of anesthesia sufficient to intubate the animal is required to enable open-mouthed restraint for visualization and to suppress the gag reflex. Thiobarbiturates, propofol, and ketamine–diazepam (Valium), with or without premedication, have all been described for this purpose. One small prospective study showed that thiopental was preferred to propofol or other sedative protocols because it exhibited the least depressive effect on laryngeal motion.[5] A case series of dogs undergoing flexible laryngoscopy by way of a transnasal approach reported that the use of premedication only (acepromazine and an opioid) was adequate to facilitate nasal passage of the endoscope without an induction agent, thus avoiding the issue of respiratory depression by the induction agent.[4] However, the use of opioids may also depress the cough reflex sufficient to interfere with assessment of laryngeal function.[3] A prospective study found that doxapram (2.2 mg/kg, intravenous) increased intrinsic laryngeal motion in dogs that were premedicated with an opioid and induced with propofol, thus facilitating evaluation of laryngeal function.[6]

From the oral approach, the clinician depresses the epiglottis and/or restrains the soft palate from obstructing the view; this manipulation is not needed from the transnasal approach, which may allow the larynx to be evaluated in a more normal anatomic position. The larynx is inspected for color, structure, symmetry, motion, and the presence of masses or foreign bodies; however, the most common reason for laryngoscopy is suspicion of laryngeal dysfunction. In the normal animal, both arytenoid cartilages abduct equally with each inspiration. Absence of abduction of the arytenoid cartilages upon inspiration confirms the diagnosis of laryngeal paralysis. Care must be taken to ensure that arytenoid function is evaluated during the inspiratory phase of respiration because passive paradoxic movement of the arytenoids may be observed during forceful expiration and may be mistaken for true abduction. This may be achieved by an assistant verbalizing the phase of breathing, for example, "in" and "out," while the larynx is monitored. Unilateral or bilateral laryngeal paresis or paralysis occurs in dogs and rarely in cats.[2] Most dogs with laryngeal paralysis also have erythematous vocal folds because of turbulent airflow; in cats, the paralyzed laryngeal folds may appear soft or floppy, and may seem to flutter upon expiration.[3] The laryngospasm that occurs in cats associated with any manipulation of the pharyngeal area can be confusing and must not be interpreted as laryngeal paralysis. One investigator notes that the arytenoids in such cats should normally appear firm and tight and will be observed to move after a sufficient period of waiting. The same investigator suggests that particularly challenging cases may be clarified by closing the sedated cat's mouth over a rigid laryngoscope to minimize stimulation of laryngospasm for a longer period of observation.[3]

Regardless of the anesthetic protocol or the approach chosen, it is essential to avoid an erroneous diagnosis of laryngeal paralysis based on shallow breathing as a result of too deep a plane of sedation, inadvertent pressure on the glottis by the blade of the laryngoscope, and/or positioning the neck at an acute angle that obscures visualization of both vocal folds.[1,2] Though suspicion of laryngeal paralysis is the most common reason that laryngoscopy is performed, it is critical that the clinician has knowledge of less common laryngeal disease processes, such as laryngitis, laryngeal masses, or laryngeal collapse. Laryngeal collapse is a loss of cartilage rigidity that allows medial deviation of the components of the larynx and is generally secondary to chronic upper airway obstruction in brachycephalic dogs. Thorough knowledge of normal anatomy and the appearance of normal arytenoid movement enables recognition of these anatomic changes. Surgical management of laryngeal paralysis and laryngeal collapse are significantly different and have been reviewed.[7]

TRANSTRACHEAL WASH

Cooperative dogs of medium size or larger are candidates for transtracheal wash (TTW), whereas smaller dogs, cats, or uncooperative patients of either species are better suited to endotracheal wash (ETW). Although consensus does not exist on a size cut-off for TTW, this author prefers ETW for dogs less than 7 kg and for all cats. Both washing techniques are used to obtain diagnostic samples from nonspecific regions of the proximal respiratory tree, although TTW can also obtain material from deeper regions, as the animal is able to cough during the procedure. In either case, infectious, inflammatory, and neoplastic conditions may be diagnosed.[8]

TTW is performed with the patient awake, which is one of its advantages. An awake dog coughs during the procedure, increasing the likelihood of obtaining diagnostic material from the airways. TTW is contraindicated in fractious or aggressive dogs because of the risk for tracheal or handler injury. Dyspneic dogs or dogs that may progress to a dyspneic state when stressed also have better diagnostic alternatives than TTW.[8]

Comfortably, but firmly, restrain the patient in sternal recumbency, with its nose slightly elevated. The TTW procedure takes several minutes, and the patient will need to maintain this position. Lidocaine (2%) is infused intradermally and subcutaneously for local anesthesia and requires at least 10 minutes to take effect. Clip a wide square over the ventral neck, encompassing the larynx and proximal cervical trachea, and prepare it using sterile gloves and surgical scrub (eg, 4% chlorhexidine).

Several catheters have been used, but this author prefers a long through-the-needle, intravenous catheter (eg, Venocath, Abbott Labs, Abbott Park, Ilinois or Intracath, BD, Franklin Lakes, New Jersey), for its ease and speed of use and the ability to remove the sharp needle from the trachea once the catheter has been introduced. After the skin is prepared, palpate the cricothyroid ligament with a gloved finger as a half-circular, slightly yielding depression distal to the firm and prominent thyroid cartilage. With the bevel facing ventrally, introduce the needle through the skin and through the cricothyroid ligament, into the tracheal lumen. Resistance, followed by a light pop, is felt as the cricothyroid ligament is crossed, at which point the advancement of the needle is stopped. Gently angle the tip of the needle down approximately 45° and advance the catheter through the needle. If the needle is properly positioned, the catheter feeds easily down the open tracheal lumen. Resistance suggests that the needle bevel has not fully crossed the ligament or has abutted the dorsal (far) wall of the trachea. Close examination and careful repositioning should allow correction of this situation. Feed the catheter until it locks into the needle hub, then extract the needle and snap its guard into place, leaving only the soft, flexible catheter in the airway.

Attach a preloaded syringe containing 5 to 20 mL of sterile (nonbacteriostatic) 0.9% saline to the catheter and flush the fluid into the trachea. The volume of fluid is proportional to patient size, although there is no consensus as to the dose of TTW fluid per body weight. Typically, the dog begins to cough promptly, but if not, it can be encouraged to do so by coupage. Meanwhile, use the syringe to aspirate fluid and secretions back though the catheter. Air will also be aspirated, usually in far greater proportion than fluid; air must be evacuated from the syringe to avoid losing any portion of the fluid sample, or additional syringes must be used to continue aspiration. Expect to retrieve a tenth or less of the infused volume. Infuse additional aliquots of saline and recover samples until adequate diagnostic material is obtained.

Gently and firmly extract the catheter from the trachea, and apply a sterile non-adherent gauze square with firm pressure covered by a light neck wrap, which is left in place for the next several hours. Monitor the dog for development of subcutaneous emphysema, which is rare, and usually self-limiting. Samples obtained by TTW are suitable for cytology and culture, as described later, or for special diagnostics, such as polymerase chain reaction (PCR), virus isolation, or specific antigen assays.

Endotracheal Wash

ETW is a similar technique used in patients in whom TTW is not appropriate. ETW requires a brief period of general anesthesia sufficient to permit intubation. Intubation of the patient is achieved with a sterile endotracheal tube by an operator wearing sterile gloves with the patient in sternal or lateral recumbency (with the more severely affected side down). Feed a sterile, red rubber catheter down the endotracheal tube, and use syringes preloaded with sterile (nonbacteriostatic) 0.9% saline to infuse and aspirate as described earlier.

Disadvantages to this procedure include the inability of the patient to cough, which reduces yield, and the possibility of oropharyngeal contamination at the time of intubation. Material collected by ETW is suitable for cytology, culture, or special diagnostics; cytology should always be closely evaluated for evidence of oropharyngeal contamination, such as the presence of *Simonsiella* species organisms, or squamous epithelial cells, as described in more detail below.

TRACHEOBRONCHOSCOPY

Dogs and cats are candidates for tracheobronchoscopy if acute or chronic clinical signs of cough, hemoptysis, stridor, or dyspnea have not been diagnosed by other means.[1,9] Animals with primarily vascular lesions, focal pulmonary lesions, or diffuse interstitial disease may be less likely to benefit from direct visualization of the airways by tracheobronchoscopy. Tracheobronchoscopy is useful in animals with suspected, or confirmed, tracheal collapse, because it provides additional information regarding the severity, extent, and dynamic aspects of collapse that may not be appreciated with radiographic or fluoroscopic examination.[2] Tracheobronchoscopy is most valuable when coupled with BAL for diseases located in the small airways or alveoli.[10] Caution is indicated in patients with severe respiratory compromise, or patients considered high-risk for general anesthesia. In two studies in cats, bronchoscopy and guided sampling diagnosed inflammatory airway disease, bacterial and fungal pneumonia, neoplasia, pulmonary fibrosis, and bronchial collapse/bronchiectasis.[11,12] Comprehensive descriptions of veterinary tracheobronchoscopy equipment and its care and use have been reported.[9,10,13–16]

Anesthesia

The subject of anesthesia for bronchoscopic procedures has been thoroughly addressed, and the reader is referred to these publications for greater detail.[13,17,18] A few points bear special mention.

General anesthesia is required, and most clinicians prefer inhalant anesthesia for all but the smallest patients. In two reviews of bronchoscopy in cats, anesthesia consisted of propofol infusion, and oxygen was provided by jet ventilation.[11,12] Similarly, two reviews of bronchoscopy in dogs described injectable anesthesia without intubation, regardless of the size of the dog.[15,19]

When using inhalant anesthesia, the largest possible, sterile, endotracheal tube is used for intubation. Use a sterile T- or Y-shaped adapter, containing a soft, snug port for the passage of the bronchoscope to connect the endotracheal tube to the anesthetic breathing system. Place a mouth gag to prevent endoscope trauma, should the plane of anesthesia decrease for any reason.

In cats and some small dogs, the bronchoscope may occlude the lumen of an appropriate-sized endotracheal tube sufficiently to prevent simultaneous adequate delivery of oxygen and gas anesthesia. If injectable agents are not chosen in these cases, the examination and diagnostic sampling must be performed in several brief segments. During visual examination, while the bronchoscope occludes the lumen of the endotracheal tube, deliver oxygen to the patient through the working channel of the bronchoscope.[13] After a brief inspection, remove the endoscope and resume anesthetic gas delivery, and repeat the procedure to complete the examination. Diagnostic sampling can be performed on subsequent passes of the endoscope down the endotracheal tube. Other clinicians prefer to anesthetize and stabilize the patient with inhaled agents, then extubate immediately before the bronchoscopic examination, maintaining anesthesia with injectable agents. Application of a topical anesthetic, such as lidocaine, may help decrease laryngospasm in cats any time a bronchoscope is passed in the absence of an endotracheal tube.

In addition to anesthetic premedications, some clinicians advocate premedication with a bronchodilator, such as aminophylline or terbutaline, because of a concern for bronchoconstriction induced by the procedure.[10] Preliminary evidence from a retrospective study in cats suggested that pretreatment with terbutaline for 12 to 24 hours before bronchoscopy reduced the rate of complications seen after bronchoscopy and BAL.[11]

Tracheobronchoscopic Anatomy and Appearance

Canine tracheobronchial anatomy has been described, and a schematic system of nomenclature for reports of bronchoscopic findings has been reported (**Fig. 1**).[20] Most authors accept this anatomic map as a general guideline for use in the cat, and subtle differences in feline anatomy have been described.[15,21] The extent to which lobar, segmental, and subsegmental bronchi can be visualized in a given patient depends upon patient size, bronchoscope diameter and length, and clinician skill. In all but the smallest patients, the endoscope passes easily through the trachea, carina, and right and left mainstem bronchi, and the origins of the lobar bronchi can be visualized. In the largest patients, a bronchoscope of adequate length can be passed through lobar, segmental, and some subsegmental bronchi.

Normal tracheobronchial mucosa is light pink and moist with scant secretions. Submucosal vessels are easily visible, as are tracheal cartilage rings. The dorsal tracheal membrane is visible as a tight, narrow band of tissue firmly fixed to the dorsal wall. The carina appears as a sharp division, and the normal entrances to the right and left principal bronchi are smooth, round, and well defined. Branching of the airways quickly becomes more complex, and size may preclude entry of the endoscope, but all normal branches seen have a well-defined, round, patent orifice.

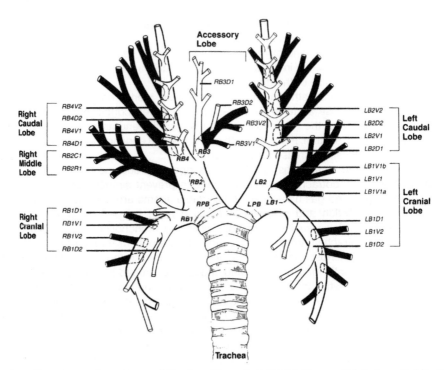

Fig. 1. Bronchoscopic anatomy of the dog. (*From* Amis TC, McKiernan BC. Systematic identification of endobronchial anatomy during bronchoscopy in the dog. Am J Vet Res 1986;47(12):2655; with permission.)

Examination Procedure

With the dog or cat positioned in sternal recumbency, gently pass the bronchoscope through the respiratory tract, and do not use force at any time. Endoscopists familiar with gastrointestinal endoscopy will note the difference between that system, where insufflation is required to maintain lumen patency and the walls yield to pressure as the endoscope passes around turns, and the rigid, patent respiratory tract.

Examine the respiratory tree in a systematic manner, passing down the trachea, into the right mainstem bronchus and each of its subsequent branches to the limit of length of the endoscope or diameter of the airway lumen. Retract the endoscope and enter the opposite bronchus and repeat the procedure. Should the clinician lose track of the anatomic location of the scope at any time, back the endoscope to the level of the carina and resume the examination from there to provide reorientation. Throughout the examination, patency, color and character of mucosa, presence and character of secretions, and presence and location of masses or foreign bodies are observed and recorded. Clinician experience plays a substantial role in the ability to recognize normal versus abnormal tissue.[13] If properly equipped, digital photographs should be made of areas of interest. A standardized reporting form, including an anatomic diagram shown earlier, helps to maintain a consistent approach in each patient. Only after the visual examination is complete should sampling be done.

SAMPLE COLLECTION
Bronchoalveolar Lavage

BAL samples cells and material from the small airways and alveoli, deeper than typically obtained with TTW or ETW. Samples can be obtained from a specific anatomic region, if warranted by endoscopic findings, or from a random selection of sites. Some clinicians do not find BAL reliable for focal lesions because of the difficulty in reliably accessing a specific site and consider it more appropriate for diffuse lower airway disease.[22] BAL is typically performed after visual examination but before any other sampling procedures, such as brushing or biopsy, to avoid altering the results by the presence of iatrogenic hemorrhage.

Pass the endoscope down the trachea toward the region of interest until it wedges in the smallest bronchus that accommodates it. Because overall length of the bronchoscope can limit distal reach, sometimes the tip of the endoscope must be directed into the nearest branching airway at each subsequent level. This may direct the bronchoscope away from the region of interest; however, if there is diffuse disease, wedge the endoscope as distal as possible on the right side, and repeat the procedure on the left.

Successful collection of diagnostic fluid samples requires infusion of an adequate volume of fluid and tight fit of the bronchoscope into the regional bronchus to facilitate recovery of a high percentage of that fluid. However, as is the case with TTW/ETW, there is debate surrounding the ideal dose of fluid for BAL, although most authors do agree that at least two bolus infusions per site should be performed. One author used at least two boluses, 25 mL each, per site of interest in most dogs. For dogs less than 8 kg and all cats, he used at least four boluses, 10 mL each, per site of interest.[10] In a report on dogs, another author used a total volume of 15 to 75 mL per dog, divided into two or more aliquots.[23] In a retrospective study of 68 cats, the mean volume of fluid infused for BAL ranged from 2.62 to 5.05 mL/kg. This corresponded to the use of 5- or 10-mL aliquots, at the preference of the attending clinician.[11] Another feline retrospective used 5- to 20-mL aliquots for BAL, according to the preference of the attending clinician.[12] In dogs, recovery of 40% to 50% of infusate has been reported.[23] In the retrospective of 68 cats, 50% to 75% of the infused fluid was recovered, and the cell counts were considered adequate for cytologic evaluation in 97% of the procedures, independent of infusate volume.[11]

Once the endoscope is wedged, attach a syringe preloaded with the chosen amount of sterile (nonbacteriostatic) 0.9% saline solution to the working channel. Push the saline as a bolus and begin recovery of fluid as soon as infusion is complete. Use the same syringe to forcefully aspirate the working channel. If the bronchoscope is imperfectly wedged, air is frequently aspirated, and the syringe quickly fills with fluid and air. Use a new syringe to continue aspiration, or the original syringe may be detached and its air contents ejected into the room, taking care not to eject any portion of the recovered sample. In some cases, aspiration yields negative pressure without fluid recovery, which is presumed to be because of airway collapse in response to suction. The endoscope should be backed out very slightly if this occurs, and aspiration repeated.[10] An alternate technique used at the author's institution is to attach a suction trap to the suction port of the bronchoscope. Vacuum suction is attached to the suction trap, and the endoscope's suction feature is used to recover the infused fluid immediately after bolus injection through the working channel. In the author's hands, this allows for a greater yield on fluid recovery, without the need for repeated changing or evacuating of syringes. Especially in the case of a large patient, where the endoscope may not be completely wedged into the area of interest, the use of continuous vacuum suction seems preferable. There are anecdotal concerns of excessively forceful suction and/or disrupted cellular architecture by this technique, but to the author's knowledge, these outcomes have not been reported.

In rare instances, the endoscope will be too short to wedge into a desired region. In these instances, lavage may still be performed as described earlier, with the knowledge that the percentage of fluid recovered will be decreased. Alternatively, clinicians at the author's institution and elsewhere have used a long polytetrafluoroethylene catheter (eg, ASPC-1, Endoscopy Support Services, Brewster, New York) or polyethylene catheter,[15] fed down the working channel of the bronchoscope. Feed the tubing out the end of the endoscope and pass it further down the bronchus until resistance is felt. The tubing can be observed bronchoscopically as it is fed, but its final distal location cannot be seen or controlled. Infuse sterile saline through the catheter as described earlier, and recover the fluid by syringe aspiration. Care must be taken when sampling blindly in this manner, because of the concern that diseased airway is likely more sensitive to trauma by mild pressure.[15] Samples retrieved in this way are heavily mixed with air, but the technique does enable sampling of an otherwise unreachable area.

Samples retrieved by BAL are appropriate for cytology, culture, or special diagnostics, such as PCR, virus isolation, or specific antigen assays. Because multiple infusions are typically performed, samples are generally recovered in discrete syringes. A study evaluated cytology results based on individual samples (first to third) from a patient versus a pooled sample from that same patient and found no difference in results; pooling samples therefore seems appropriate.[24]

Bronchial Brushing

Bronchial brushing may obtain cells that are adherent to the mucosa and are not collected by BAL.[23] Perform the procedure using endoscopic brushes contained within a retractable plastic sheath. Pass the brush down the working channel to the area of interest, and advance it from the plastic sheath; drag it gently over the mucosa in the region of interest, retract it back into the sheath, and then withdraw it from the working channel. Material retrieved by bronchial brushing is suitable for culture or cytology. For culture, the brush end may be transected with sterile scissors and placed into a sterile container for transport to the laboratory, or the brush end may be swirled through culture medium, taking care not to contaminate the medium with the plastic sheath. For cytology, gently roll the brush across glass slides.

Biopsy

Biopsy, using specially designed endoscopic biopsy forceps, is indicated for nodules or masses within the airway lumen.[25] Sample collection is technically difficult because the rigid anatomy of the airways orients the endoscope and biopsy forceps parallel to the lesion.[15] Sample size is also limited by the size of forceps that passes through the working channel; any pieces retrieved are small and are subject to crush artifact at the time of acquisition.[25] Because of these challenges, bronchoscopic biopsy is the least commonly performed bronchoscopic diagnostic sampling technique. Multiple samples are required to assure a consistent finding, but increasing the number of samples also increases the risk of hemorrhage or perforation; an optimal number of biopsy samples has not been determined. [13,25]

SAMPLE SUBMISSION
Cytology

Fluid obtained by TTW, ETW, or BAL and material obtained by bronchial brushing are all suitable for cytologic examination. Cytologic samples may be submitted as fluid or as prepared slides, depending on the preference of the laboratory and the nature of the material obtained. Fluid submissions enable the laboratory to use cytospin techniques to concentrate low numbers of cells. When submitting samples as fluid, ethylenediaminetetraacetic acid is recommended to preserve cellular morphology.[22]

Presence of infectious agents is also evaluated by cytology, and cytologic findings are used to interpret culture results. As the tracheobronchial tree is not a sterile site in normal dogs, the cytologic finding of intracellular bacteria, particularly as a monomorphic population, is most supportive of true infection.[19,26,27] Again, the finding of *Simonsiella* organisms or squamous epithelial cells on cytology indicates oral contamination and suggests that culture results are suspect. Differences in findings among sampling techniques bear mention here, and the reader is referred to other reports for comprehensive review of normal and abnormal respiratory cytology.[22]

Transtracheal wash or endotracheal wash

Normal cytologic findings from TTW or ETW are cells that are easily washed from the proximal mucosal surface, including respiratory epithelial cells, neutrophils, eosinophils, lymphocytes or macrophages, and mucus. Cytologic descriptions should include estimated cellularity, differential counts, and morphologic descriptors of cells encountered, although precise and accurate cell counts are not possible with this technique.

It is important to recall that neutrophils, macrophages, and eosinophils are part of normal immune surveillance of the respiratory mucosa and are normally found in this site, but their relative frequencies and morphology can be informative.[1] The predominant leukocyte in most small-animal TTW/ETW is the neutrophil.[13,22] However, normal cats may have up to 25% eosinophils recovered.[15,22,27] Mucus is a normal finding on TTW/ETW cytology, but Curschmann's spirals represent inspissated mucus and small-airway obstruction.[22] Although occasional bacteria are seen in normal TTW/ETW samples, special attention should be paid to the finding of intracellular bacteria, especially if the population is monomorphic, and to the presence of fungal elements.[28] Neoplastic cells are of particular significance, although caution is warranted in discriminating between clusters of hyperplastic epithelial cells versus squamous metaplasia and true neoplasia.[1,22]

Bronchoalveolar lavage

Cytology obtained by BAL differs from TTW or ETW, in that the cells are sampled from deeper branches of the respiratory tree. In addition to morphologic description and relative cellular percentages, some clinicians perform total nucleated cell counts on samples obtained by BAL. Although normal counts have been reported, inconsistencies in fluid volumes and sample handling techniques make establishment of absolute counts controversial.[10,13,22,29]

Cellular percentages and morphology are generally considered more important than absolute counts, and relative increases in white blood cells can be seen with inflammation and infection. The alveolar macrophage is the most common cell recovered in BAL fluid, (>70%) which differs from the predominance of the neutrophil in TTW/ETW.[13,22] Surfactant (rather than mucus, as seen in TTW/ETW) is a normal finding in BAL samples and causes foaminess in the recovered fluid.[22] Diagnoses achievable by BAL, perhaps preferentially to other means, include bacterial, fungal, viral, parasitic, and protozoal (*Toxoplasma gondii*) infection, noninfectious inflammation, lymphoma, and carcinoma, but variable cell yield, location, and diseases which poorly exfoliate can limit usefulness.[10,12] A small, feline retrospective study compared the diagnosis achieved by BAL with histopathology (necropsy or lung lobectomy). The correlation between BAL and histopathology was incomplete; particularly noteworthy were cases in which neoplasia was diagnosed on histopathology, but inflammation was diagnosed on BAL. This highlights the concern that neoplastic cells may not exfoliate readily under BAL conditions, and more invasive diagnostics may need to be considered if a strong index of suspicion for neoplasia exists despite an inflammatory diagnosis from BAL.[12]

Bronchial brushing

Cytology obtained by bronchial brushing is similar to BAL, but it may include cells that would not have been easily washed free from the mucosa. In a study that compared BAL to bronchial brushing in dogs with chronic cough, brushing was found to yield an increased number of neutrophils compared with BAL. Additionally, in five dogs where neutrophil counts in BAL fluid were considered normal, four samples obtained by brushing revealed neutrophilic inflammation.[23] This finding suggested that brushing may be more sensitive than BAL for inflammatory states because brushing detected the white blood cells that were adherent to bronchial walls in addition to those that readily washed free.

Culture

The tracheobronchial tree is not a sterile site in normal dogs, and bacteria of unknown clinical significance are reported in dogs with chronic bronchitis.[13,19,26,27] For this reason, some clinicians recommend quantitative or semiquantitative bacterial cultures of BAL fluid, and it has been reported that greater than 10^4 colony forming units (CFU)/mL (or grown from primary culture) represents true infection whereas less than 10^3 CFU/mL (or grown from subculture) represents contamination.[1,13] However, many clinicians still perform only routine cultures because of financial or logistic concerns.[10] Because BAL also dilutes the organisms present (if any) by a variable amount, even quantitative cultures need to be interpreted in light of cytologic and clinical findings. In addition to standard aerobic bacterial cultures, mycobacterial cultures, particularly in cats, and fungal cultures in properly equipped laboratories, may also be indicated.

BAL is often reserved for patients who have failed therapeutic trials; as such, BAL fluid is commonly collected from animals that are receiving or have recently received antimicrobial therapy. Even antimicrobial agents that have failed to resolve the clinical signs may exist in high enough concentration to inhibit in vitro culture, so some clinicians recommend that BAL samples always be cultured from enrichment broth.[10]

A study described quantitative bacterial cultures and cytologic examination of fluid obtained by BAL in dogs. A cut-off point of 1.7×10^3 CFU/mL or more yielded a sensitivity of 86% and specificity of 100% for the diagnosis of lower respiratory tract infection. The presence of intracellular bacteria on cytologic examination as an additional diagnostic criterion changed these values slightly, yielding a sensitivity of 87% and a specificity of 97%.[19]

COMPLICATIONS

Complications associated with airway endoscopic and diagnostic procedures are rare and include worsening of cough or induction of bronchospasm, especially in cats with hyperreactive airways.[15] Complications reported in a retrospective study in cats included hemoglobin desaturation during the procedure (12 of 68 cats), prolonged anesthetic recovery (4 cats), requirement for supplemental oxygenation following the procedure (4 cats), and pneumothorax (2 cats); all of these cats survived to discharge.[11] In the same study, however, 4 cats were euthanized after bronchoscopy because of inability to alleviate the underlying cause of respiratory distress (1 cat) or lack of recovery of spontaneous ventilation after anesthesia (3 cats).[11] Factors such as signalment, duration of clinical signs before bronchoscopy, and final diagnosis did not predict the occurrence of complications.[11] In any animal with chronic respiratory disease that has become dependent on exaggerated respiratory effort to maintain airway patency, there is a concern that respiratory suppression (by sedation or anesthesia) may permit collapse of diseased airways.[15]

SUMMARY

Flexible endoscopy is a valuable diagnostic approach to the upper and lower respiratory tract, because it allows direct visualization and sample collection. Techniques requiring a range of specialized equipment and varying levels of experience have been developed to access and evaluate each anatomic region. Familiarity with appropriate indications for each procedure and normal appearance, cytology, and culture results from each region will enhance diagnostic success.

REFERENCES

1. Padrid P. Pulmonary diagnostics. Vet Clin North Am Small Anim Pract 2000;30(6): 1187–206.
2. Bjorling D, McAnulty J, Swainson S. Surgically treatable upper respiratory disorders. Vet Clin North Am Small Anim Pract 2000;30(6):1227–51.
3. Noone KE. Rhinoscopy, pharyngoscopy, and laryngoscopy. Vet Clin North Am Small Anim Pract 2001;31(4):671–89.
4. Radlinsky MG, Mason DE, Hodgson D. Transnasal laryngoscopy for the diagnosis of laryngeal paralysis in dogs. J Am Anim Hosp Assoc 2004;40(3):211–5.
5. Jackson AM, Tobias K, Long C, et al. Effects of various anesthetic agents on laryngeal motion during laryngoscopy in normal dogs. Vet Surg 2004;33(2): 102–6.
6. Miller CJ, McKiernan BC, Pace J, et al. The effects of doxapram hydrochloride (Dopram-V) on laryngeal function in healthy dogs. J Vet Intern Med 2002;16(5): 524–8.
7. Fossum TW. Small animal surgery. St. Louis: Mosby/Elsevier; 2007.
8. Syring RS. Tracheal washes. In: King LG, editor. Textbook of respiratory disease in dogs and cats. St. Louis: WB Saunders; 2004. p. 128–34.
9. Kuehn NF, Hess RS. Bronchoscopy. In: King LG, editor. Textbook of respiratory disease in dogs and cats. St. Louis: WB Saunders; 2004. p. 112–8.
10. Hawkins EC. Bronchoalveolar lavage. In: King LG, editor. Textbook of respiratory disease in dogs and cats. St. Louis: WB Saunders; 2004. p. 118–27.
11. Johnson LR, Drazenovich TL. Flexible bronchoscopy and bronchoalveolar lavage in 68 cats (2001–2006). J Vet Intern Med 2007;21(2):219–25.
12. Norris CR, Griffey SM, Samii VF, et al. Thoracic radiography, bronchoalveolar lavage cytopathology, and pulmonary parenchymal histopathology: a comparison of diagnostic results in 11 cats. J Am Anim Hosp Assoc 2002;38(4):337–45.
13. McKiernan BC. Bronchoscopy. In: McCarthy TC, editor. Veterinary endoscopy for the small animal practitioner. St. Louis: Elsevier Saunders; 2005. p. 201–27.
14. Chamness CJ. Endoscopic instrumentation. In: Tams TR, editor. Small animal endoscopy. St. Louis: Mosby; 1999. p. 1–16.
15. Johnson L. Small animal bronchoscopy. Vet Clin North Am Small Anim Pract 2001;31(4):691–705.

16. Rha JY, Mahony O. Bronchoscopy in small animal medicine: Indications, instrumentation, and techniques. Clin Tech Small Anim Pract 1999;14(4):207–12.
17. Gross ME, Dodam JR, Faunt KK. Anesthetic considerations for endoscopy. In: McCarthy TC, editor. Veterinary endoscopy for the small animal practitioner. St. Louis: Elsevier Saunders; 2005. p. 21–9.
18. Johnson LR, Drazenovich TL. Flexible bronchoscopy and bronchoalveolar lavage in the cat: procedure and outcome (2001–2006). J Vet Intern Med 2006;20(3):746.
19. Peeters DE, McKiernan BC, Weisiger RM, et al. Quantitative bacterial cultures and cytological examination of bronchoalveolar lavage specimens in dogs. J Vet Intern Med 2000;14(5):534–41.
20. Amis TC, McKiernan BC. Systematic identification of endobronchial anatomy during bronchoscopy in the dog. Am J Vet Res 1986;47(12):2649–57.
21. Caccamo R, Twedt DC, Buracco P, et al. Endoscopic bronchial anatomy in the cat. J Feline Med Surg 2007;9(2):140–9.
22. Andreasen CB. Bronchoalveolar lavage. Vet Clin North Am Small Anim Pract 2003;33(1):69–88.
23. Hawkins EC, Rogala AR, Large EE, et al. Cellular composition of bronchial brushings obtained from healthy dogs and dogs with chronic cough and cytologic composition of bronchoalveolar lavage fluid obtained from dogs with chronic cough. Am J Vet Res 2006;67(1):160–7.
24. Hawkins EC, Kennedystoskopf S, Levy J, et al. Cytologic characterization of bronchoalveolar lavage fluid collected through an endotracheal tube in cats. Am J Vet Res 1994;55(6):795–802.
25. Bauer TG. Lung biopsy. Vet Clin North Am Small Anim Pract 2000;30(6):1207–26.
26. McKiernan BC, Smith AR, Kissil M. Bacterial isolates from the lower trachea of clinically healthy dogs. J Am Anim Hosp Assoc 1984;20(1):139–42.
27. Padrid PA, Feldman BF, Funk K, et al. Cytologic, microbiologic, and biochemical analysis of bronchoalveolar lavage fluid obtained from 24 healthy cats. Am J Vet Res 1991;52(8):1300–7.
28. Crews LJ, Feeney DA, Jessen CR, et al. Utility of diagnostic tests for and medical treatment of pulmonary blastomycosis in dogs: 125 cases (1989–2006). J Am Vet Med Assoc 2008;232(2):222–7.
29. Hawkins EC, Denicola DB, Kuehn NF. Bronchoalveolar lavage in the evaluation of pulmonary disease in the dog and cat—state-of-the-art. J Vet Intern Med 1990;4(5):267–74.

Flexible Endoscopy in Small Animals

Steffen Sum, DVM, Cynthia R. Ward, VMD, PhD*

KEYWORDS

- Fiberscope • Endoscope components • Esophagoscopy
- Gastroduodenoscopy • Enteroscopy • Colonoscopy
- Patient preparation

Flexible endoscopy is a valuable tool for the diagnosis of many small animal digestive tract diseases. This article provides a basic introduction to small animal gastrointestinal endoscopy including its diagnostic advantages as well as its limitations and complications. Although proficiency in endoscopic techniques can only be obtained through many hours of practice, this article should also encourage and stimulate the novice endoscopist. The introduction contains information about indications for gastrointestinal endoscopy, required equipment, patient preparation, and tips for the manipulation of the fiberscope. The introduction is followed by a section about the examination of different sections of the digestive tract and their most common disorders. Small animal gastrointestinal endoscopy is in demand and this trend is expected to continue to grow. There are good reasons for this: many pet owners are already aware of the clinical benefits and availability of flexible endoscopy; the veterinarian has the opportunity to establish a diagnosis earlier in the disease process, to increase revenue, and enhance professional enjoyment.

Flexible endoscopy is a minimally invasive technique using a fiberscope to visualize the gastrointestinal lumen and, particularly, collect tissue or fluid samples for further analysis such as histopathology or bacterial culture. Over the last 3 decades, flexible endoscopy has evolved to become an important diagnostic option and sometimes even a therapeutic solution. Flexible endoscopy is one of the most important techniques to evaluate patients with gastrointestinal signs. Common indications are described in **Box 1**. Frequently, occult disease is diagnosed by using endoscopic techniques. Other diagnostic tests such as blood chemistry, (contrast) radiography, and gastrointestinal ultrasound may not be sensitive or specific enough to clearly identify the disorder. In some cases an endoscopic procedure may be therapeutic as with placement of a gastrointestinal feeding tube (eg, percutaneous endoscopic gastrostomy [PEG] tube) or even curative such as with the treatment of esophageal strictures

College of Veterinary Medicine, Department of Small Animal Medicine and Surgery, University of Georgia, 501 DW Brooks Drive, Athens, GA 30602, USA
* Corresponding author.
E-mail address: cward@vet.uga.edu (C.R. Ward).

Vet Clin Small Anim 39 (2009) 881–902
doi:10.1016/j.cvsm.2009.05.009
0195-5616/09/$ – see front matter © 2009 Published by Elsevier Inc.
vetsmall.theclinics.com

Box 1
Common clinical signs indicating flexible endoscopy
Abdominal pain
Anorexia
Constipation
Diarrhea
Dyschezia
Dysphagia
Flatulence
Hematemesis
Hematochezia
Hypersalivation
Melena
Mucoid feces
Nausea
Regurgitation
Retching
Tenesmus
Vomiting
Weight loss

or the removal of gastrointestinal foreign bodies. Endoscopy of the alimentary tract can be divided into upper gastrointestinal tract endoscopy (endoscopy of the mouth, esophagus, stomach, and duodenum) and lower gastrointestinal tract endoscopy (endoscopy of the rectum, colon, cecum, ileum).

ENDOSCOPIC EQUIPMENT

The basic equipment to perform small animal gastrointestinal endoscopy consists of a flexible fiber-optic endoscope and a light source. A high-intensity halogen or xenon light bulb produces cold light. Most modern units also contain an air pump and a water flush pump. The pumps enable the examiner to insufflate air, thereby displacing the mucosa from the distal viewing lens for better visualization. The water is mainly used for cleaning the viewing lens or flushing debris away from the region of interest. Bundles of glass fibers within the endoscope are used for illumination as well as for transporting the picture of the object to the proximal end where it can be viewed through an ocular lens (eyepiece). Special lens systems magnify the image along its path. A video camera can be attached to the eyepiece to forward the image to a monitor. The monitor enables the investigator to comfortably observe the magnified image and to share it with other people. Modern flexible endoscopes already contain a video microchip in the handpiece and thus are called video endoscopes. The electronic signals of the video chip are transmitted to a video processor, which then forwards the images to the monitor. This video system provides superior optical quality but is also more expensive. Modern units are fully digital, which further improves the image quality. Ideally, an electronic data storage system (eg, CD burner, hard drive) is connected to the image processor or monitor so that examination findings can be documented and stored for later reviews. Additional external suction pumps or vacuum lines are used to deflate organs or remove fluid from the patient's gastrointestinal tract during the examination.

COMPONENTS OF AN ENDOSCOPE

The basic flexible fiber-optic endoscope consists of three major components: the handpiece, the insertion tube, and the umbilical cord (**Fig. 1**).

The handpiece of the endoscope (**Fig. 2**) contains the eyepiece for visualization as well as the main control mechanisms. There is a larger up/down dial and a smaller left/right dial to navigate the scope within the gastrointestinal tract. Most endoscopes have locks to fix these wheels. In addition, there are two knobs attached to the handpiece: a suction valve (usually marked red) and an air/water valve (usually marked blue). Depression of the suction valve provides aspiration of air or fluid through the working channel. Occlusion of the blue valve (air/water valve) causes air to pass through the insertion tube. This air is used for insufflation. Depression of the same valve causes a nozzle to spray water against the viewing lens for cleaning.

The flexible insertion tube is the part of the fiberscope that is inserted into the patient's gastrointestinal tract for examination. It contains the fiber optics for imaging and illumination, the mechanics to flex the scope in different directions, and two channels. The air/water channel provides air for insufflation and water for cleaning purposes, whereas the working channel is used to pass instruments (eg, biopsy forceps) and to remove air or fluid by suction. Most of these components can be viewed at the tip of the fiberscope (**Fig. 3**). The tip of the endoscope is highly flexible and can be deflected by rotation of the two dials at the handpiece: up and down as well as left and right. Modern fiberscopes used for gastroduodenoscopy offer at least 90° of flexion in three planes and 180° in one plane (**Fig. 4**).

The umbilical cord is so named because it connects the endoscope to all the supporting modules. The external light source submits light through the fiber-optics and pumps provide air, water, or vacuum suction through this line. In the video endoscope, cables and electronics to transmit the electronic signals from the video chip to the external processor are also contained within the umbilical cord.

TYPES OF FLEXIBLE ENDOSCOPES

Modern fiberscopes are similar in basic construction and consist of the components mentioned earlier. They mainly differ in length and diameter of the insertion tube,

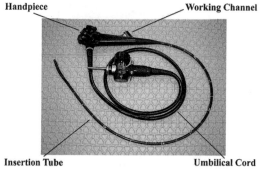

Handpiece   Working Channel

Insertion Tube   Umbilical Cord

Fig. 1. Fiberscope components.

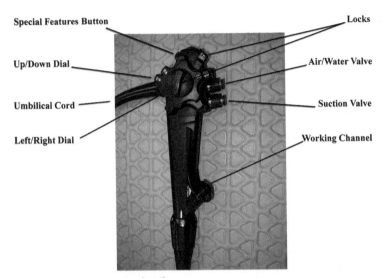

Special Features Button

Locks

Up/Down Dial

Air/Water Valve

Umbilical Cord

Suction Valve

Left/Right Dial

Working Channel

Fig. 2. Handpiece components in detail.

flexibility, optical and mechanical quality, as well as price. It is impossible to build one endoscope for all applications because the different procedures have different requirements. Before an endoscope is purchased, its intended use should be considered. Most fiberscopes are manufactured for the human medicine market, their name reflecting their main field of application (eg, bronchoscope, gastroscope, urethroscope, **Fig. 5**). Generally, the smaller the diameter and the greater the length, the poorer the optical quality of the fiberscope. A small diameter insertion tube usually also has a small diameter working channel, which limits the size of the biopsy instruments that can be passed. This limitation will affect sample size and, as a result, quality. Working channel size should be large enough to pass forceps of 2.4 mm (7 Fr) or larger to obtain diagnostic samples.[1] Most currently available human gastrointestinal endoscopes have an insertion tube length of 100 to 110 cm and diameters ranging from 8 to 12 mm. Unfortunately, although easily available, some of these fiberscopes are not the

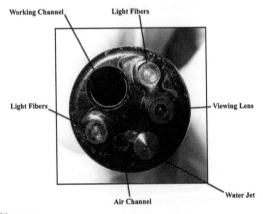

Working Channel

Light Fibers

Light Fibers

Viewing Lens

Air Channel

Water Jet

Fig. 3. Tip of the fiberscope.

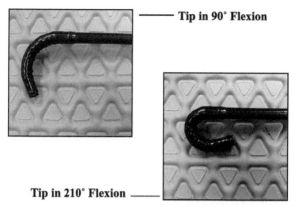

Tip in 90° Flexion

Tip in 210° Flexion

Fig. 4. Flexion of the fiberscope tip.

best choice for most small animal practitioners: a 12-mm diameter insertion tube is often too big to be passed through the pylorus of smaller dogs and cats, and a 110-cm insertion tube length may not be long enough to reach into the duodenum of large dogs. Fortunately, some manufacturers have begun to produce more versatile scopes for the veterinary market. They have forward-viewing optics with insertion tubes of smaller diameter (7–9 mm) and lengths of 120–160 cm. Their working channels are large enough to accept biopsy forceps of 2.4 mm (7 Fr) or larger, which will provide tissue samples of diagnostic adequacy if the right technique is used.[1] These types of endoscopes offer the best value for the budget-minded practitioner who wants to pursue small animal gastrointestinal endoscopy with only one fiberscope.

ENDOSCOPIC INSTRUMENTS

Numerous flexible instruments are available for use with a fiberscope. The most basic equipment consists of biopsy forceps and foreign body forceps. In addition, cytology brushes, aspiration/injection needles, and various foreign body retrieval devices (eg, slings, baskets; **Fig. 6**) can be helpful. The experienced endoscopist may even consider coagulation electrodes or laser equipment. The selected instruments must be determined to be compatible with the fiberscope to be used. Several types of

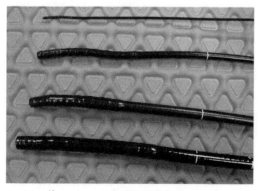

Fig. 5. Different fiberscopes (from top to bottom: 2.5-mm urethroscope; 5.9-mm broncho-scope; 8.6-mm gastroscope; 11.3-mm gastroscope).

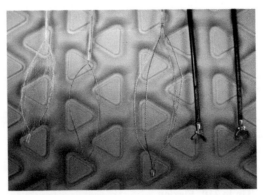

Fig. 6. Different foreign-body grasping devices (from left to right: basket; loop; wire basket; forceps with alligator jaws; forceps with 1 × 2 teeth).

biopsy forceps are available (**Fig. 7**): round or oval cups with or without alligator teeth, and with or without a central spike. Gastroenterologists often disagree as to which type of forceps provides the best samples. Biopsy forceps with spikes can prevent slippage during biopsy but may provide a less deep biopsy sample. Forceps with alligator teeth often provide the biggest samples on upper gastrointestinal tract endoscopy but smaller pieces of tissue if used for colonoscopy. A human study illustrated that although one design might be slightly superior for certain applications compared with others, most current designs are able to provide good quality samples.[2] The most important aspect is to use biopsy forceps of at least 2.4-mm diameter or larger. If smaller biopsy forceps are used, more samples might have to be taken to get a confident diagnosis. All biopsy instruments should be kept clean, sharp, and well lubricated. The samples should only be submitted to a pathologist who is experienced in evaluating small animal gastrointestinal biopsies.[3] He or she should be aware of the histopathological standards of gastrointestinal inflammation.[4]

MANIPULATION AND STORAGE OF THE FIBERSCOPE

Before the patient is anesthetized, perform a quick system check. Test all necessary functions of the endoscope and any other equipment to be used (including

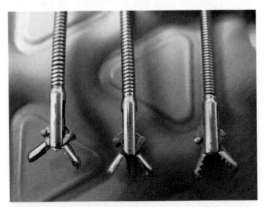

Fig. 7. Different biopsy forceps (from left to right: biopsy forceps with oval cupped jaws; biopsy forceps with oval cupped jaws and spike; biopsy forceps with toothed, oval cupped jaws).

instruments) to avoid technical problems during the endoscopic examination. Use the "one-handed technique" to manipulate the fiberscope during the following examination: hold the handpiece of the endoscope in your left hand (**Fig. 8**). Use the left thumb, index, and middle finger to rotate the dials. The tip of the left index finger manipulates the air water valve (blue knob) while the tip of the middle finger operates the suction valve (red knob). Use the right hand to advance, torque, and withdraw the insertion tube.

Alternatively, the "two-handed technique" can be used, which is usually easier for the beginner: hold the handpiece with the left hand, but use the fingers of the right hand to operate the dials and valves. Move the insertion tube in small steps using the right hand while wheel and valve adjustments are made using the same hand whenever the insertion tube is not manipulated.

After completion of the endoscopic examination, clean the fiberscope promptly following the manufacturer's recommendations. Usually, a soft wet cloth is used to remove particles and debris on the outside of the insertion tube. Then, after removing the valves at the handpiece, perform a leak test before the endoscope is submersed in water or cleaning solutions. Most newly purchased fiberscopes come with a leak test kit provided by the manufacturer. If not, a model-specific kit can be ordered. If there is leakage, the endoscope should only be superficially cleaned according to the manufacturer's specification and shipped to an authorized repair facility for service. More thorough cleaning should be avoided because it could cause water to enter the sensitive fiber-optical or electronic system resulting in major damage. If the endoscope passes the leak test, next submerge the endoscope into a cleaning solution. The detergent used must be compatible with the fiberscope (see manufacturer's recommendations). Most modern detergents contain specific enzymes that help break up protein rich particles and require a certain dwell time. Specific brushes are used to clean bigger particles from the working channel and valves. Cleaning units that pump the cleaning solution through the different channels either manually or

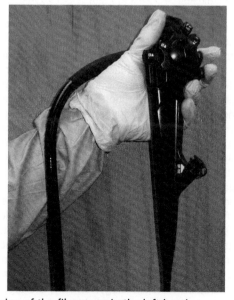

Fig. 8. Correct positioning of the fiberscope in the left hand.

automatically are available through different vendors. The last step is rinsing the outside and the channels of the fiberscope with clean water to remove the detergent and the endoscope is hung up for drying. The best way of storing a flexible endoscope is by hanging it close to the handpiece. The endoscope can be hung within a lockable cabinet to prevent theft or unauthorized usage. Styrofoam tubes (eg, used for insulation), pulled over the end of the insertion tube, can provide further protection to the fragile fiber-optics. If a fiberscope is handled correctly, cleaned properly, and stored appropriately, it should provide several years of service.

PATIENT PREPARATION, EQUIPMENT SET UP, AND COLLECTION OF SAMPLES

Fast the patient for 12 to 18 hours, and withhold water for at least 4 hours before gastroduodenoscopy. The length of fasting before colonoscopy is determined by the type of cleansing to be performed as well as the patient's overall condition. Inadequate cleansing will make the examination much more difficult and lesions could be missed. The ideal fasting period for lower gastrointestinal endoscopy is 36 to 48 hours and, water may be given up to 4 hours before anesthesia. The fasting period can often be reduced to 24 to 36 hours if oral cleansing solutions (eg, GoLYTELY, NuLYTELY) are administered. These are isotonic electrolyte solutions that promote mild osmotic diarrhea. They are manufactured for human use. Consequently, administration by stomach tube in dogs or nasoesophageal tube in cats is required in most animals. They should be given at a dose of 10 to 20 mL/kg twice on the day before the procedure and once the day of the procedure, each at least 2 hours apart. In addition, give multiple enemas before performing the colonoscopy with the last one no closer than 2 hours beforehand. For routine examination of the alimentary tract, place the patient in left lateral recumbency (**Fig. 9**) so that the pylorus is up and the duodenum can easily be entered. In this position, adjacent organs place the least pressure on the stomach. There is an exception for endoscopic gastric tube placement: place the patient in right lateral recumbency, which places the stomach adjacent to the abdominal wall, enabling the operator to push a trocar through the abdominal and gastric walls into the gastric lumen. General anesthesia is required for all these procedures, and a cuffed endotracheal tube is used to prevent aspiration. Anesthetic machinery should be set up so as not to interfere with the examination.

The endoscopist stands in front of the mouth of the patient for upper endoscopy and in front of the anus for lower endoscopy. Place a mouth gag before oral insertion of the endoscope. If video endoscopy is performed, position the monitor so that the examiner is facing the screen. This way, orientation through the endoscopic examination is easiest: downward movement of the up/down dial will move the picture on the screen downward, moving the left/right dial to the right will move the picture on the screen to the right, and so forth. Only advance the endoscope when the lumen is clearly visible. The lumen can usually be visualized if it is distended, which is achieved by the insufflation of air through the air/water valve. Sometimes, visualization is obscured due to contractions of the gastrointestinal tract. If so, the endoscopist should wait until the contraction has terminated and the surrounding tissue relaxes. Never use undue pressure to advance the fiberscope or instruments. If orientation is lost, the endoscopist should withdraw the endoscope and reorientate, then continue to move forward.

Whenever a patient undergoes gastrointestinal endoscopy and a thorough visualization has been completed, obtain tissue samples from different locations of the gastrointestinal tract. Frequently, the definitive diagnosis of chronic gastrointestinal disease is based primarily on histopathology. Usually, the bigger the samples, the better their quality. Thus, use the biggest flexible biopsy forceps that can pass through

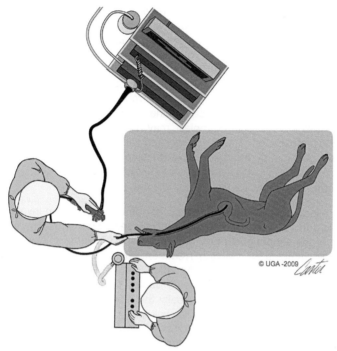

Fig. 9. Patient positioning for routine gastrointestinal endoscopy.

the working channel of the insertion tube. Extend the biopsy forceps beyond the tip of the fiberscope and advance them to the area to be sampled. Directional control is obtained by manipulating the up/down and the left/right dial. Open the forceps when they get close to the biopsy site and advance them firmly into the tissue. The cups of the forceps should be directed perpendicular to the mucosal wall or as close to perpendicular as possible. Deflating the lumen may help obtain good quality samples. The advancement of the biopsy forceps will meet some resistance from the gastrointestinal wall. Once increased resistance is met, close the forceps firmly. Withdraw the biopsy forceps to the tip of the endoscope and tear free the tissue sample using a firm steady tug. Forceful tearing or gently teasing should be avoided because it can result in damaged and distorted samples. Masses should be sampled as deeply as possible. Whenever possible, biopsies should be taken under visual control. Sometimes, the "blind biopsy technique" (without visualization) is used to obtain samples from as far down the small intestines as possible (eg, jejunum) or when taking biopsies of the ileum through the ileocolical sphincter during colonoscopy. In these circumstances, the forceps are advanced until resistance is met out of sight. Then, open the cups, grab the tissue, and withdraw the forceps.

In dogs and cats, obtain six to seven such samples of each anatomic location (ie, jejunum, duodenum, stomach).[5] Tissue samples can be submitted for routine histopathology or bacterial culture, but they can also be used for impression smear cytology, or fast tests (eg, a test for urease-splitting bacteria). If mucosal samples are to be used for histopathology, submit the samples in accordance with the histopathology laboratory's recommendations. Most laboratories prefer the use of small plastic histopathology cassettes rather than saline-moistened lens paper. The biopsy samples must be removed from the biopsy forceps with great care. Samples are best removed using a 22- to 25-gauge needle (canula) to carefully sweep the sample out of the cup of the forceps and stretch it onto the foam of a histopathology cassette. When sampling of a particular organ (eg, stomach) has been completed, close the cassette and place it into a jar with formalin. In addition, you can obtain brush cytology samples or fluid samples using an aspiration tube. Endoscopically obtained cytology results often correlate with histopathologic results in cases of neoplastic or inflammatory disease. However, because cytology generally produces results quicker than routine histopathology, a diagnosis can potentially be obtained while the patient is still under anesthesia. In addition, cytologic samples may provide useful information about bacterial flora, protozoa, or parasites associated with the mucosal surface. This information usually gets lost during processing of tissue samples for histopathology.

ESOPHAGOSCOPY

Endoscopic examination of the esophagus, esophagoscopy, is an invaluable tool in the diagnosis and treatment of esophageal disease.[6] Esophagoscopy allows direct visualization of the esophageal mucosa and the opportunity to obtain cytologic and histopathologic samples for analysis. Treatment such as balloon dilation of esophageal strictures and direct application of medications to the mucosal and submucosal surfaces are possible. Esophageal foreign bodies may be removed by esophagoscopy. Although contrast imaging is usually the diagnostic choice for investigating megaesophagus, esophageal diverticula, vascular ring anomalies, fistula, or hiatal diseases, esophagoscopy can offer additional information about the appearance of the esophageal mucosal surface so that the practitioner may offer additional treatments.[7]

Clinical signs of esophageal disease include regurgitation, dysphagia, hypersalivation, coughing, anorexia, and weight loss. Occurrence of these clinical signs may point the practitioner to esophageal disease, and esophagoscopy is warranted.

Flexible endoscopes, including fiber-optic and video, are the preferred instruments for esophagoscopy. Rigid endoscopes may be used; however, it is difficult to obtain a full examination of the esophagus due to the abnormal angles the esophagus must adopt to accommodate the rigid endoscope. It is less likely that the entire esophagus may be viewed. In addition, there is an increased chance of esophageal perforation if a rigid endoscope is used. Should an esophageal foreign body be present requiring a rigid instrument for removal, one can be passed next to the flexible endoscope.

Patient Preparation

General anesthesia is required for esophagoscopy. Animals should be intubated with a well-inflated tracheal cuff to prevent aspiration. Copious amounts of food and fluid may be present in the esophagus if motility is abnormal. Ideally, fast the animal for at least 12 hours. Esophageal contrast studies, especially those using barium, should be avoided before esophagoscopy, as barium can obstruct proper visualization of the esophagus. If barium or another contrast agent has been used, the practitioner should wait 24 hours before esophagoscopy. If remnants of the contrast agent remain, thoroughly lavage the esophagus to remove as much contrast as possible to allow visualization of the esophagus.

Esophagoscopic Procedure

The esophagus can be visualized with the animal in right or left lateral recumbancy. Usually left lateral recumbancy is preferred because gastroduodenoscopy often follows esophagoscopy. A mouth gag is placed before insertion of the endoscope.

The cervical esophagus is entered right behind the larynx. Air insufflation should begin immediately. It may take a few minutes for the esophagus to become dilated with air. An assistant may hold off the esophagus just distal to the larynx to prevent air escape through the mouth. After the esophagus is dilated, the endoscope is passed, keeping the esophageal lumen centered in the field of view. Air insufflation should continue for the entire procedure so that the esophagus is dilated. Esophageal diverticula are more easily identified in a dilated esophagus. Initial passing of the endoscope should occur slowly to allow for full visualization of the esophagus, as only with the first passing can the practitioner be sure there has been no iatrogenic damage to the esophagus by the endoscope. The esophageal examination is complete when the lower esophageal sphincter is visualized. The practitioner should image any abnormalities if possible.

The normal dog esophageal mucosa is pink and glistening. Dog breeds, such as the chow chow, that have pigmented oral mucosa may have patches of pigmented mucosa. Extraesophageal structures can be seen imprinted on the flaccid esophagus, most notably the pulsation of the aortic arch as the endoscope approaches the base of the heart. The esophagus of the cat is slightly different in appearance in that circular rings formed by the mucosa are present in the distal esophagus.

Routine biopsies of the esophagus are usually not obtained. Healthy esophageal mucosa is tough and biopsies are hard to obtain. However, if a mucosal lesion or mass is present, samples should be submitted for cytology or histopathology. These can be obtained with biopsy forceps or cytology brushes.

Esophageal Stricture

Strictures of the esophagus can occur from gastroesophageal reflux, foreign body passage, trauma, neoplasia, esophageal surgery, ingestion of irritants or medications, or even severe esophagitis.[8–10] Often, esophageal strictures are diagnosed following a general anesthetic procedure because of reflux of gastric contents. These lesions can be devastating depending on the severity and chronicity of the stricture. Clinical signs are compatible with those of esophageal disease including regurgitation, coughing, anorexia, weight loss, and aspiration pneumonia.

Strictures can be easily visualized by esophagoscopy as a ring of fibrous tissue that narrows the lumen of the esophagus. Full insufflation of the esophagus will aid in the visualization. Often the area around the stricture is erythematous due to the esophageal damage causing the lesion. It is often helpful to obtain contrast imaging before esophagoscopy so that the extent of the stricture can be visualized. In addition, the practitioner may be able to choose the right size endoscope to pass through the stricture, although in some cases it is not possible.

Esophageal strictures can be treated with balloon dilation.[11] If held at a specific size, the balloon provides radial forces that dilate the stricture in a centrifugal manner. Balloon catheters are available in many sizes, and one catheter may be dilated to different sizes depending on the amount of saline infused into the balloon. Although most catheters are designed for single use, they can be cleaned and sterilized for repeated use. Always check the balloon integrity before the procedure.

Balloon catheters can be inserted through the biopsy channel; however, they are more easily passed next to the endoscope so that they can be visualized. The balloon is passed until the center of it is in the center of the stricture. The balloon is dilated according to the manufacturers specifications and held in place for 90 to 120 seconds. This procedure may be repeated several times under the same anesthetic event. Often there will be bleeding associated with the ballooning. To lessen the chance of re-stricture, injectible triamcinolone may be injected submucosally around the dilated stricture site. Specialized injection needles may be passed through the endoscope, and a submucosal bleb can be directly visualized following the injection. Usually, 0.1 to 0.2 mL of triamcinolone is placed in several sites around the stricture. Balloon dilation should be repeated twice per week, as necessary, for up to 12 procedures.

GASTROSCOPY

After ruling out food sensitivity, parasites, and obstruction, gastroscopy is the obvious choice for small animal patients with chronic upper gastrointestinal signs. Whenever gastroscopy is performed, duodenoscopy should be performed also. In most cases with chronic disease, duodenoscopy actually provides the diagnosis.

In addition to provide visual documentation of the gastrointestinal lumen, gastro-duodenoscopy enables the examiner to obtain tissue or fluid samples for further diagnostics. Furthermore, it can be curative as in the case of foreign body removal, or therapeutic as with placement of feeding tubes (eg, PEG tube or J-tube). However, if tissue samples are taken with flexible biopsy forceps, they usually consist of the most internal mucosal layers (ie, lamina epithelialis, lamina propria mucosae). Thus, the limitation of gastroduodenoscopy is the inability to diagnose submucosal disease as well as gastrointestinal motility disorders. Depending on the size of the patient and the length and diameter of the available endoscope, the insertion tube may not be passed far enough to reach the lesion. Another limiting factor is the size or shape of gastrointestinal foreign bodies. These sometimes are just too big or smooth to be grasped by foreign body forceps, loops, or baskets making them impossible to be removed by endoscopy.

Complications associated with gastroduodenoscopy are rare. All the procedures listed in this article do require general anesthesia with its associated risks. The most common complication is that the inexperienced examiner may insufflate too much air into the stomach causing overdistention. Overdistention can lead to hypotension and decreased respiratory function of the patient. It is easily prevented by constant repeated checks by abdominal palpation and thorough monitoring of blood pressure and breathing of the patient. Perforation of the gastrointestinal tract is extremely rare as long as the endoscopist takes care not to use too much force.

Endoscopic Technique and Normal Findings

The endoscopist should develop a protocol and always examine the different areas within the stomach in the same sequence to make sure that an area is not missed. Different examiners use different protocols, especially for performing the retroversion maneuver. To pass the lower esophageal sphincter, center the tip of the fiberscope at the gastroesophageal orifice. This positioning is usually accomplished by deflecting the tip of the endoscope approximately 30° to the left with a simultaneous slight upwards deflection as the lower esophageal sphincter is passed. Short puffs of air while gently pushing can facilitate the passage. There should be only minor resistance to advancing the endoscope into the stomach. On entry, the tip of the endoscope will now face the greater curvature with its rugal folds. In most dogs, the stomach walls will still be partially or completely collapsed. At this point, the endoscopist should pause and insufflate air to distend the stomach, which will flatten the rugal folds enabling evaluation of all of the mucosa in this area (**Fig. 10**). Care should be taken to not over-inflate the stomach. Overinflation can cause cardiopulmonary compromise and gastric mucosal ischemia, and makes the passage of the endoscope through the pylorus more difficult. Gradually advance the fiberscope following the rugal folds along the greater curvature until the antrum is reached. Only minor direction changes are usually needed to provide a panoramic view. By moving the tip slightly upwards, visualize the

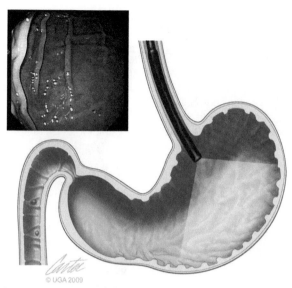

Fig. 10. View and positioning of the fiberscope on entering the stomach.

incisura angularis (**Fig. 11**). This distinctive fold extends from the lesser curvature and is an important landmark that separates the body of the stomach from the antrum. The examiner can appreciate the view of two tunnels divided by the incisura. The upper tunnel is the gastric body whereas the lower tunnel is the antrum. If the up/down dial is now further turned counterclockwise up to its maximum, the tip will pass the incisura and point back to the fundus and cardia. This technique is also called the "retroversion maneuver" or "J-maneuver" (**Fig. 12**), in which the examiner can see the fiberscope as it passes the lower esophageal sphincter. By applying mild torque clockwise and counterclockwise to the insertion tube, next evaluate the fundic area adjacent to the cardia. Withdrawing the fiberscope once this view is attained will pull the endoscope tip closer to the cardia. Because of the smaller size of the feline stomach, an en face view of the incisura is not always achieved. Instead, start the retroversion maneuver when the tip of the endoscope is in the mid body area. Finally, straighten the tip again and advance into the antrum. In dogs, antral peristaltic waves may be observed when approaching the antrum. These are seen as round symmetric rings that form in the proximal antrum and sweep toward the pylorus. They occur in a frequency of three to four contractions per minute. Antral peristaltic waves are rarely observed in cats unless prokinetic drugs have been administered. At the end of the antral canal, the pylorus should come into view (**Fig. 13**). It usually is closed during the contractions.

If the patient has been properly fasted, the stomach should be free of food and fluid. The normal gastric mucosa is smooth and has a reddish pink color. Overall, it is redder than the esophageal mucosa. Overinsufflation can cause some areas to have a patchy whitish appearance. If air is insufflated, the stomach should distend easily and the rugal folds should flatten. Usually, there are no folds in the antrum. Antral folds can result from mucosal hypertrophy, polyps, chronic inflammation, or neoplasia. The antrum should also be free of bile. Gastric biopsies should be taken after the fiberscope has been advanced through the pylorus and the duodenum has been thoroughly examined and biopsies taken.

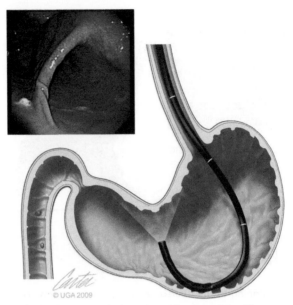

Fig. 11. View of angular incisura angularis and positioning of the fiberscope.

GASTRIC DISEASES
Gastritis

In small animals, acute or chronic inflammation of the gastric mucosa is common. Possible causes include dietary indiscretion, infection, drugs or toxins, and gastric foreign bodies. Especially in acute gastritis, the etiologic cause is not always

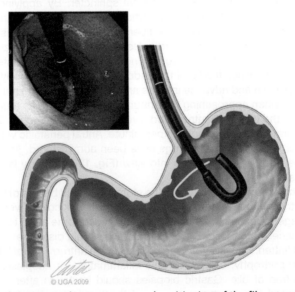

Fig. 12. View during retroversion maneuver and positioning of the fiberscope (insertion tube can be seen as it passes through the cardia).

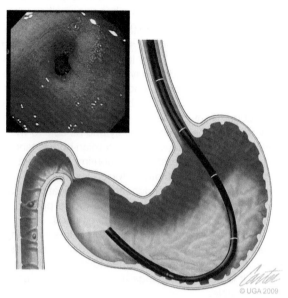

Fig. 13. View of pylorus and positioning of the fiberscope.

identifiable. Mucosal hyperemia is probably the least reliable clue to gastric disease because color changes often represent vascular changes but not mucosal disease. Better clues are mucosal irregularity (eg, ulcers), mucosal friability, rugae folds that fail to flatten with gastric insufflations, and prominent lymph follicles. Sometimes, refluxed bile is present in the antrum, or active duodenogastric reflux can be observed during the endoscopy.

Ollulanus tricuspis and *Physeloptera* sp are parasites that can cause gastritis in small animals. *Olluolanus tricuspis* infection is found in cats. Microfilariae of this parasite are approximately 0.7 mm in length and can be identified by examining gastric fluid under the microscope using low-power magnification. *Physeloptera* sp causes gastritis in dogs and cats. Infected individuals are often presented for chronic vomiting. Adult forms of this parasite can be found in the stomach or the duodenum by direct visualization during endoscopy. This visualization is important because this parasite's eggs are often missed on routine fecal flotation.

Helicobacter are spiral-shaped or curved, sometimes coccoid gram-negative bacteria that inhabit the glands, parietal cells, and mucus of the stomach.[12] *Helicobacter jejuni* is known to cause chronic lymphocytic-plasmacytic gastritis in humans. Some species of this spirochete are believed to cause disease in cats and dogs. The pathogenicity and the clinical significance of this organism in regard to chronic gastritis in small animals are still not fully understood.[13] A substantial number of clinically healthy dogs and most clinically healthy cats are infected with *Helicobacter*-like organisms.[14–16] *Helicobacter*-associated gastritis can be characterized by the presence of ulcers or prominent lymph follicles. Spirochetes can be found on histopathology or brush cytology of gastric mucosal samples and are suggestive of infection. Because *Helicobacter* sp is able to split urease, fast tests can be used for preliminary diagnosis. A diagnosis of lymphocytic gastritis due to *Helicobacter* infection should be made only after other possible causes have been ruled out.

Atrophic gastritis is a rare chronic inflammatory disease characterized by diffuse lesions particularly in the body and fundus. The mucosa seems to be thinner and paler compared with other locations within the stomach. It is mainly described in Norwegian Lundehunds and seems to be associated with gastric adenocarcinoma.[17,18]

Hypertrophic gastritis is characterized by a macroscopic thickening of the gastric mucosa with large rugal convulsions. Focal lesions occur at the pyloric antrum and are mainly seen in geriatric toy breeds. They may cause delayed gastric emptying. Diffuse hypertrophy is rare and has been reported in basenjis and in a boxer.[19–21]

Gastric foreign bodies are a common problem in small animal medicine and are often found in young dogs. Many of these can be removed by endoscopy. Limiting factors are the ability to grasp the object securely and be able to withdraw it through the lower esophageal sphincter. Because gastric foreign bodies tend to move quickly and pass through the pylorus, it is essential to confirm the object's location radiographically before the animal is anesthetized for endoscopy. The presence of food or fluid in the stomach can make the endoscopic identification of a gastric foreign body much more difficult. If a delay is not harmful to the patient, the endoscopic procedure can be postponed until the stomach has emptied.

If the patient is placed in left lateral recumbency, most freely moving gastric foreign bodies will be located in the fundus just below the cardia. Thus, most foreign bodies can be seen just after the endoscope enters the stomach or during the retroversion maneuver. Sometimes it is helpful to change the position of the patient to make the foreign body more accessible.

The first challenge is to grasp the foreign body. Using the appropriate grasping instrument often determines the success or failure of the procedure. Whereas small flat objects (eg, coins) usually can be best grabbed with pointed grasping forceps, larger round objects (eg, golf balls) are best immobilized and retrieved by putting a net over them. Ideally, an array of different foreign body retrieval tools should be available to the endoscopist.

The second challenge is to retract the immobilized object through the powerful lower esophageal sphincter. Withdraw the foreign body with gradually increasing force and straighten the endoscope tip to prevent loss of the object. Often it is helpful to place a large-diameter stomach tube over the insertion tube before entering the stomach and grasping the foreign body. Then the stomach tube dilates the lower esophageal sphincter and is withdrawn along with the fiberscope before the immobilized foreign body passes.

After the successful removal of a gastrointestinal foreign body, always reevaluate the stomach and intestines endoscopically to make sure that all foreign bodies have been retrieved and that no major damage to any organs has occurred. Biopsies of the stomach and small intestines should be routinely taken to rule out concurrent disease and to make sure that the foreign body is the cause of the patient's presenting complaints and not simply an incidental finding.

Gastric Ulceration

Gastric ulcers are grossly detectable mucosal defects within the stomach. There are two types commonly seen in small animals: single large, deep ulcers surrounded by a firm raised wall and sometimes containing a fibrin plug (resembling moon craters), and multiple, small, more superficial ulcers. Ulcers may be actively bleeding on examination or the visualized blood may have a "coffee-ground" appearance due to partial digestion. Biopsies must not be taken from the center of a big ulcer so as not to cause penetration of the gastric wall. Furthermore, histopathology of the center of a big ulcer usually only reveals necrotic tissue and is rarely useful diagnostically. Instead, biopsies should be taken from the margins of the ulcer, as well as adjacent, more normal-looking mucosa. Diseases associated with the formation of gastric ulcers are neoplastic disease (eg, adenocarcinoma), *Helicobacter* sp infection, and gastric-acid hypersecretion, which occurs with gastrinomas and mast-cell tumors.

Gastric Neoplasia

The two most common malignant gastric neoplasms in small animal medicine are lymphosarcoma in cats and adenocarcinoma in dogs. Lymphosarcoma often presents as a large masslike growth in the body of the stomach. Occasionally, it is more of a diffuse lesion and can be identified by prominent rugal folds that fail to flatten during insufflation. Ulceration can be associated with gastric lymphoma. Gastric adenocarcinoma is rare and the most common sites are the antrum and the lesser curvature, followed by the greater curvature.[22] Frequently, mucosal ulceration is also present. If the gastric adenocarcinoma is mainly submucosal, the stomach may resist distention and the rugal folds may resist flattening during insufflation. To obtain deeper, submucosal tissue samples, the endoscopist will have to take repeated biopsies from the same spot, to dig deep enough into the gastric wall.

The most common benign gastric neoplasms are mucosal polyps and leiomyomas. Leiomyomas are usually smooth submucosal masses, and are often located close to the lower esophageal sphincter. They are often incidental findings unless they cause obstruction.

Intestinal Endoscopy

Indications for intestinal endoscopy, also called enteroscopy, are detailed in **Box 1**. Whenever gastroscopy is performed, the endoscopist should also evaluate the upper small intestine to complete the examination. Enteroscopy is the least invasive means to obtain small intestinal biopsy samples useful for diagnosing several important diseases such as the various types of inflammatory bowel disease. Limitations of intestinal endoscopy include difficulty passing the fiberscope through the pylorus and the limited length of the insertion tube, which most often can only reach as far as the duodenum.

Endoscopic Technique and Normal Findings

For the beginner, advancing the fiberscope through the pylorus into the duodenum is often perceived as the most difficult and frustrating aspect of gastroduodenoscopy. As mentioned earlier, entering the pylorus is most easily achieved with the patient in left lateral position. In rare cases, a temporary rotation of the patient into dorsal recumbency might be helpful. Overdistention of the patient's stomach should be avoided. It is essential to keep the opening of the pyloric sphincter exactly centered in the endoscope's field of view. Keeping the view centered requires continuous corrections while the endoscope is patiently advanced with steady moderate pressure. Most often, precise alignment and slow advancement will be rewarded with entry into the pylorus. If multiple trials fail, a second technique can be tried in which the examiner directs biopsy forceps into the pyloric opening using them as a guide. The insertion tube is then moved over the forceps until the tip enters the pyloric canal. This technique often leads to iatrogenic erosions in the proximal duodenum, which has to be remembered consequently when small superficial ulcerations are detected in this area. Once within the pyloric canal, short puffs of insufflated air can help widen the lumen making it easier to advance the fiberscope. At the end of the pyloric canal, the tip of the endoscope usually runs into the wall of the most proximal duodenum, which is characterized by a sharp right and downward turn of about 90° in most cats and dogs. If this occurs, the lumen of the duodenum will cease to be visible because the viewing lens of the endoscope will become stuck in intestinal mucosa. This phenomenon is called pink-out, and requires redirecting the tip of the endoscope to the right and down. Further insufflation of air often will distend the lumen far enough to be visualized. The position of the tip is corrected as necessary and the endoscope is further advanced toward the lumen. Further gentle advancement will usually provide a tunnel view of the descending duodenum (**Fig. 14**). Usually, insufflation is required to distend the walls. Advance the insertion tube as far as possible. Then the examiner should start taking mucosal biopsies all the way back to the pylorus.

The duodenal mucosa is paler than the gastric mucosa. The color is whitish pink to whitish cream. It also has a rougher, grainy texture that is due to thousands of villi. This granular appearance fades if the lumen is distended by insufflation of air. Peyer's patches appear as whitish, well-demarcated circular indentations along the intestinal wall. A minor amount of bile-colored fluid within the lumen is normal. The duodenal papillae can usually be identified as small, raised, circular buttons that are redder in color than the adjacent tissue. There are two in the dog: the major duodenal papilla (opening of the common bile duct), originating approximately 3 to 5 cm from the pylorus, and the minor duodenal papilla (opening of the pancreatic duct) identifiable about 2 cm caudal of the major papilla and more dorsal. Cats have only one duodenal papilla containing the opening of a duct that leads to the common bile duct and the pancreatic duct.

INTESTINAL DISEASES
Endoparasites

Metazoic parasites such as ascarids and *Physeloptera* sp can be identified on visualization in the duodenal lumen. Giardiasis in dogs can be diagnosed by intestinal fluid aspiration and microscopic cytologic evaluation. This technique often fails in cats because *Giardia* organisms usually colonize the distal small intestines. Fecal tests by smear and flotation can be negative for these pathogens because eggs may only get shed intermittently.

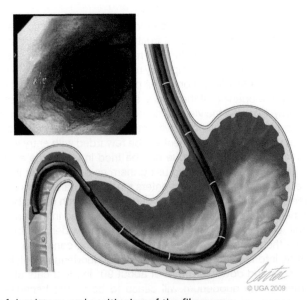

© UGA 2009

Fig. 14. View of duodenum and positioning of the fiberscope.

Small Intestinal Bacterial Overgrowth

Small intestinal bacterial overgrowth (SIBO) is characterized by an uncontrolled increase in the number of bacteria in the upper small intestines. In small animal medicine, bacterial overgrowth is a poorly understood condition.[23,24] The quality and quantity of the small intestinal bacterial flora depends on many factors including host genetics, gastrointestinal motility, production of gastric acid and digestive enzymes, diet, and the mucosal immune system. The condition can be of primary idiopathic nature, as seen in young German shepherd dogs, or, more often, a sequela of other gastrointestinal disease.[25–28] Because the idiopathic form usually responds to antibiotic therapy, some investigators have recommended that this condition be renamed antibiotic-responsive diarrhea (ARD).[29]

The gold standard for diagnosing SIBO is quantification of bacterial numbers from duodenal fluid culture obtained after an 8-hour fast. In dogs, more than 10^5 colony forming units (CFU) per milliliter are considered abnormal.[25] Normal cats can have higher counts, up to 10^8 CFU/mL. Duodenal fluid can be obtained using endoscopic aspiration through sterile tubes.[30] Care should be taken to prevent oral contamination or dilution of the duodenal juice with water flush. Atropine application during anesthesia should be avoided because it may decrease gastrointestinal secretion. However, the collection of duodenal juice has been replaced by less invasive and cumbersome methods, mainly by determination of cobalamin and folate in the serum of the patient. In patients with SIBO, serum folate is increased due to bacterial synthesis, whereas serum cobalamin is decreased due to bacterial binding in the intestinal lumen.[31] Because the same changes are seen in individuals with exocrine pancreatic insufficiency, serum trypsinlike immunoreactivity (TLI) concentration should be measured beforehand to rule out this disease.

Lymphangiectasia

Lymphangiectasia is a common disorder of unknown cause characterized by marked dilatation of the intestinal mucosal and submucosal lymphatics. It is commonly seen in basenjis, Yorkshire terriers, and Norwegian lundehunds, and is a major cause for protein-losing enteropathy. Impaired intestinal lymph drainage leads to stasis of chyle in the dilated lacteals and lymphatics of the intestinal wall and mesentery. Consequently, the lacteals leak or rupture and seep protein-rich lymph into the intestinal lumen. Along with protein, lymphocytes and fat are lost and lead to the usual biochemical abnormalities (panhypoproteinemia, lymphopenia, hypocholesterolemia, and hypocalcemia due to vitamin D and calcium malabsorption). Other causes of protein-losing enteropathy, such as severe inflammatory bowel disease, intestinal lymphosarcoma, and histoplasmosis, have to be excluded before making a final diagnosis. On endoscopy, the villi appear swollen and have whitish glistening appearance, and this can be enhanced by adding fat (eg, vegetable oil) to the last meal before enteroscopy. Sometimes, endoscopic biopsies may not be deep enough to diagnose this disease because submucosal lymph vessels cannot be reached. In these cases, full thickness biopsies of the duodenum or jejunum can be obtained by laparoscopy or laparotomy.

Idiopathic Inflammatory Bowel Disease

Idiopathic inflammatory bowel disease (IBD) is a common cause of chronic gastrointestinal signs in small animals. The exact cause of IBD is unknown. Host genetic susceptibility, the mucosal immune system, and environmental factors (eg, intestinal microflora) contribute to the development of the disease. IBD is a collective term for a group of disorders that are classified by the type of inflammatory cell infiltrate within the mucosa and, sometimes, deeper layers. Lymphocyic-plasmacytic, lymphocytic, eosinophilic, neutrophilic, and granulomatous types can be differentiated histologically. On endoscopy, a nodular irregular mucosa can often be visualized. Changes in color can be manifold from a pale grayish white to a hyperemic dark pink. Often, the mucosa is friable and bleeds easily after manipulation. Due to this increased friability, mucosal samples obtained by endoscopy are often larger than normal. Granulomatous IBD is regional and commonly carries a poor prognosis. Usually, masslike thickenings are visible in the colon and ileum and may cause obstruction. Mucosal rigidity and ulceration are other findings associated with this disease.

Intestinal Neoplasia

Intestinal cancer is uncommon in small animals but can be life-threatening. Nonlymphomatous small intestinal tumors include polyps, adenoma, adenocarcinoma, leiomyoma, leimyosarcoma, carcinoid, sarcoma, fibrosarcoma, plasma-cell tumor, and mast-cell tumors.[22] Focal neoplastic lesions are often characterized by mucosal irregularity and ulceration as well as narrowing of the luminal diameter. They may cause intestinal obstruction. Intestinal lymphoma can be either focal or diffuse. Diffuse intestinal lymphoma often results in an irregular, friable mucosa that is similar in appearance to IBD.

Other Findings

Other abnormalities observed during small intestinal endoscopy include intestinal ulceration, intestinal foreign bodies, intussusception, and fungal disease. Intestinal ulceration may be associated with nonsteroidal anti-inflammatory drug therapy or increased gastric acid production (eg, gastrinoma).

COLONOSCOPY

Endoscopic examination of the colon, colonoscopy, may be performed using rigid or flexible endoscopes.[32] Flexible endoscopes provide the advantage of allowing visualization of the entire colon with minimal risk of iatrogenic damage.

Indications for colonoscopy include those animals exhibiting primarily large bowel or rectal disease. Typically these animals have failed food trials or antibiotic therapy or some sort of a mass lesion is suspected. Although structural colonic abnormalities can be diagnosed using contrast radiographic techniques, colonoscopy is essential for visualization biopsy of the mucosal surfaces.

Proper patient preparation is essential for an optimal colonoscopic examination. For this the colon should be as clean as possible. Food should be withheld for 24 to 48 hours before the procedure. Oral colonic lavage solutions as described previously can be used.[33] However, they can be hard to administer and aspiration of the lavage solutions can have severe complications. They are also not appropriate in cats. Multiple warm water enemas can be effective in cleaning out the colon. They can be given at 1- to 2-hour intervals until the water exiting the rectum is clear. Routinely three to four enemas are given the night before and two to three the morning of colonoscopy. The last enema should be given no later than 2 hours before the procedure to avoid excess fluid in the colon. Care should be taken during the enema procedure in cats so that instillation of excess amounts of fluid does not cause vomiting.

General anesthesia is required to thoroughly visualize the entire colon during colonoscopy. The patient is placed in left lateral recumbency. A digital rectal examination is often performed before the procedure to make sure there are no strictures or impediments to the passage of the endoscope. The finger can also be used to guide insertion of the endoscope. The endoscope is inserted 1 to 2 cm into the rectum. Air is insufflated while an assistant closes the anus around the endoscope to prevent air escaping. After the colon is insufflated, the endoscope is slowly passed taking care to note any mucosal abnormalities. The endoscope should be centered in the colon for the best visualization. Normal colonic mucosa is easily distended and is glistening, smooth, and pink in color.

The endoscope is passed the length of the colon, gently navigating the colonic flexures until the ileocolic valve is seen. The cecum is a blind pouch next to the valve. As the ileocolic valve is sometimes open, the cecum can be mistaken for that structure and the endoscopist may become frustrated at the blind ending of the cecum. The cecum should be thoroughly visualized for any abnormalities.

Biopsies should be obtained from any abnormal areas of the colon. Should the colon appear visually normal, routine biopsies should be taken from various sites. In our hospital, six to eight biopsies are taken along the various part of the colon.

REFERENCES

1. Danesh BJ, Burke M, Newman J, et al. Comparison of weight, depth, and diagnostic adequacy of specimens obtained with 16 different biopsy forceps designed for upper gastrointestinal endoscopy. Gut 1985;26:227–31.
2. Woods KL, Anand BS, Cole RA, et al. Influence of endoscopic biopsy forceps characteristics on tissue specimens: results of a prospective randomized study. Gastrointest Endosc 1999;49:177–83.
3. Willard MD, Jergens AE, Duncan RB, et al. Interobserver variation among histopathologic evaluations of intestinal tissues from dogs and cats. J Am Vet Med Assoc 2002;220:1177–82.
4. Day MJ, Bilzer T, Mansell J, et al. Histopathological standards for the diagnosis of gastrointestinal inflammation in endoscopic biopsy samples from the dog and cat: a report from the World Small Animal Veterinary Association Gastrointestinal Standardization Group. J Comp Pathol 2008;138(Suppl 1):S1–43.
5. Willard MD, Mansell J, Fosgate GT, et al. Effect of sample quality on the sensitivity of endoscopic biopsy for detecting gastric and duodenal lesions in dogs and cats. J Vet Intern Med 2008;22:1084–9.
6. Gualtieri M. Esophagoscopy. Vet Clin North Am Small Anim Pract 2001;31: 605–30, vii.
7. Nawrocki MA, Mackin AJ, McLaughlin R, et al. Fluoroscopic and endoscopic localization of an esophagobronchial fistula in a dog. J Am Anim Hosp Assoc 2003;39:257–61.
8. Beatty JA, Swift N, Foster DJ, et al. Suspected clindamycin-associated oesophageal injury in cats: five cases. J Feline Med Surg 2006;8:412–9.
9. Glazer A, Walters P. Esophagitis and esophageal strictures. Compend Contin Educ Vet 2008;30:281–92.
10. Leib MS, Sartor LL. Esophageal foreign body obstruction caused by a dental chew treat in 31 dogs (2000–2006). J Am Vet Med Assoc 2008;232:1021–5.
11. Harai BH, Johnson SE, Sherding RG. Endoscopically guided balloon dilatation of benign esophageal strictures in 6 cats and 7 dogs. J Vet Intern Med 1995;9: 332–5.
12. Fox JG, Lee A. The role of Helicobacter species in newly recognized gastrointestinal tract diseases of animals. Lab Anim Sci 1997;47:222–55.

13. Neiger R, Simpson KW. *Helicobacter* infection in dogs and cats: facts and fiction. J Vet Intern Med 2000;14:125–33.
14. Happonen I, Saari S, Castren L, et al. Occurrence and topographical mapping of gastric *Helicobacter*-like organisms and their association with histological changes in apparently healthy dogs and cats. Zentralbl Veterinarmed A 1996; 43:305–15.
15. Hermanns W, Kregel K, Breuer W, et al. *Helicobacter*-like organisms: histopathological examination of gastric biopsies from dogs and cats. J Comp Pathol 1995; 112:307–18.
16. Geyer C, Colbatzky F, Lechner J, et al. Occurrence of spiral-shaped bacteria in gastric biopsies of dogs and cats. Vet Rec 1993;133:18–9.
17. Qvigstad G, Kolbjornsen O, Skancke E, et al. Gastric neuroendocrine carcinoma associated with atrophic gastritis in the Norwegian Lundehund. J Comp Pathol 2008;139:194–201.
18. Berghoff N, Ruaux CG, Steiner JM, et al. Gastroenteropathy in Norwegian Lundehunds. Compend Contin Educ Vet 2007;29:456–65, 468–70 [quiz 470–451].
19. Krunngen HJ. Giant hypertrophic gastritis of Basenji dogs. Vet Pathol 1977;14: 19–28.
20. MacLachlan NJ, Breitschwerdt EB, Chambers JM, et al. Gastroenteritis of Basenji dogs. Vet Pathol 1988;25:36–41.
21. van der Gaag I, Happe RP, Wolvekamp WT. A boxer dog with chronic hypertrophic gastritis resembling Menetrier's disease in man. Vet Pathol 1976;13:172–85.
22. Morrison WB. Cancer in dogs and cats. 2nd edition. Jackson (WY): Teton NewMedia; 2002. 528–9.
23. Johnston KL. Small intestinal bacterial overgrowth. Vet Clin North Am Small Anim Pract 1999;29:523–50, vii.
24. Willard MD, Simpson RB, Fossum TW, et al. Characterization of naturally developing small intestinal bacterial overgrowth in 16 German shepherd dogs. J Am Vet Med Assoc 1994;204:1201–6.
25. Williams DA, Batt RM, McLean L. Bacterial overgrowth in the duodenum of dogs with exocrine pancreatic insufficiency. J Am Vet Med Assoc 1987;191:201–6.
26. Batt RM, Needham JR, Carter MW. Bacterial overgrowth associated with a naturally occurring enteropathy in the German shepherd dog. Res Vet Sci 1983;35: 42–6.
27. Panish JF. Experimental blind loop steatorrhea. Gastroenterology 1963;45:394–9.
28. Rutgers HC, Batt RM, Elwood CM, et al. Small intestinal bacterial overgrowth in dogs with chronic intestinal disease. J Am Vet Med Assoc 1995;206:187–93.
29. Hall EJ, Simpson KW. Diseases of the small intestine. In: Ettinger SJ, Feldman EC, editors. Textbook of veterinary internal medicine. 5th edition. Philadelphia: Saunders; 2000. p. 1223–5.
30. Papasouliotis K, Sparkes AH, Werrett G, et al. Assessment of the bacterial flora of the proximal part of the small intestine in healthy cats, and the effect of sample collection method. Am J Vet Res 1998;59:48–51.
31. Batt RM, Morgan JO. Role of serum folate and vitamin B12 concentrations in the differentiation of small intestinal abnormalities in the dog. Res Vet Sci 1982;32: 17–22.
32. Willard MD. Colonoscopy, proctoscopy, and ileoscopy. Vet Clin North Am Small Anim Pract 2001;31:657–69, viii.
33. Burrows CF. Evaluation of a colonic lavage solution to prepare the colon of the dog for colonoscopy. J Am Vet Med Assoc 1989;195:1719–21.

Gastrointestinal Laparoscopy in Small Animals

Lynetta J. Freeman, DVM, MS

KEYWORDS

• Laparoscopy • Gastrointestinal • Small animals • Dog • Cat

Minimally invasive surgery (MIS) is becoming more widely adopted in veterinary medicine. The purpose of this article is to review the current status and application of laparoscopic surgery involving the gastrointestinal tract in small animals.

LIGATION OF VASCULAR RING ANOMALY

Although it is technically feasible to perform MIS procedures in the esophagus and these procedures are widely applied in human surgery, only one procedure has been adopted in veterinary medicine: ligation of the vascular ring anomaly persistent right aortic arch (PRAA). The benefits of the procedure include improved operative visualization and faster recovery from surgery. In 2001, minimally invasive surgery was reported by Dr. Eric Monnet as being used to treat a vascular ring anomaly in a puppy with PRAA and two other animals subsequently underwent surgery.[1] Selective ventilation of the right lung was performed to create a working space in the left hemothorax. Three-milliliter syringes were used as ports placed in the third and fifth intercostal spaces for insertion of a 5-mm telescope and dissecting forceps. A lung retractor was positioned from a port in the seventh intercostal space to enable the left cranial lung lobe to be retracted caudally. Dissection of the ligamentum arteriosum was performed, and clips were placed before transection of the ligament. Dissection was continued to remove all constricting fibers around the esophagus. The esophagus was dilated and repeat endoscopy confirmed release of the esophageal stricture. The animal made an uneventful postoperative recovery. Since then, Dr. Monnet has performed several other procedures successfully using the 5-mm LigaSure LAP bipolar electrocautery device (LigaSure, Valleylab, Boulder, Colorado) and converted one to an open procedure because of the presence of a double aortic arch. A complete review of this procedure is available in a separate article in this issue.

Ligation of the ligamentum arteriosum to treat PRAA is usually performed in young animals and is challenging because of a small optical cavity, dissection in and around

Department of Veterinary Clinical Sciences, Purdue University School of Veterinary Medicine, 625 Harrison Street, West Lafayette, IN 47907, USA
E-mail address: ljfreema@purdue.edu

Vet Clin Small Anim 39 (2009) 903–924
doi:10.1016/j.cvsm.2009.05.002
0195-5616/09/$ – see front matter © 2009 Elsevier Inc. All rights reserved.

the great vessels, and performing surgery on a moving target. As with open thoracotomy, surgical movements must be carefully coordinated with actions from the anesthesiologist. Because these operations are uncommon, it can be difficult to accumulate a large case series to evaluate outcomes.

Recently, there have been two large case series in human surgery. One of them, from surgeons at Emory University, reported on 13 children undergoing thoracoscopic-assisted surgery for vascular ring anomalies.[2] In this study, 9 patients had a PRAA with an aberrant left subclavian artery, and 4 had a double aortic arch with an atretic segment. The diagnosis was confirmed before surgery with MR or CT guided arteriography and three-dimensional reconstruction of the images. The patients were positioned in right lateral recumbency, and a Veress needle was used to insufflate the thoracic cavity with CO_2 to between 5 and 10 mmHg to provide exposure. Three ports were inserted, and dissection was performed using clips for ligation of the ligaments. The operative time ranged from 46 to 122 minutes (mean 70 minutes). One patient was converted to open thoracotomy because of a large double aortic arch. All of the patients recovered and their clinical signs were alleviated. Surgeons from the Children's Hospital at the Harvard Medical School reported 15 children who underwent robotic-assisted thoracoscopy.[3] Nine had patent ductus arteriosus, and 6 had vascular ring anomalies (four PRAA and 2 double aortic arch). The camera port was placed in the fifth intercostal space, and working ports were placed in the third and sixth intercostal spaces. The instruments were connected to the Da Vinci surgical robot, and the surgeon performed the dissection from a console workstation in the operating room. Stated benefits of the robotic assistance were three-dimensional visualization, the ability to use articulated or "wristed" instruments, fine tremor control, and motion scaling for precise dissection.[3] Several patients were excluded from the study because they were too small to allow the system to be used. Of 15 subjects undergoing surgery, 14 were successfully completed, and 1 was converted to an open thoracotomy because of adhesions from previous surgery. The group at Emory then reported a comparison of thoracoscopic-assisted surgery to open thoracotomy.[4] Twenty-nine children, 25 with PRAA and 4 with double aortic arch, had either attempted thoracoscopic-assisted surgery (n = 14) or open surgery (n = 15). The thoracoscopic approach was successful in 14. Two were converted to open thoracotomy. Operative times, intensive care unit stay, and hospitalization times were similar for the two approaches.

Although the da Vinci surgical system seems to offer distinct advantages for thoracoscopic procedures, robotic assistance application in animals will be limited by size and economics. Thoracoscopic correction of vascular ring anomalies should be performed by those with considerable experience in thoracic surgery. Current application is limited to patients with either a PRAA with ligamentum arteriosum or in those having atresia of a segment of a double aortic arch. When the vessel is patent, open surgery is preferred to ensure control of hemorrhage.

EXPLORATORY LAPAROSCOPY

In veterinary medicine, exploratory laparoscopy is performed when the findings can prevent unnecessary celiotomy or change the treatment course to result in an improved postoperative outcome for the animal. This decision is difficult and is left to the surgeon's judgment. Staging laparoscopy is performed after preoperative diagnostic tests fail to provide a satisfactory answer regarding the diagnosis or prognosis of an animal's condition. One benefit of staging laparoscopy is the excellent visualization of vascular changes in tissue to identify unsuspected metastatic disease.

This benefit, along with the ability to easily obtain material for cytology, culture, and biopsy, and the opportunity to observe for post biopsy hemorrhage or leakage, makes laparoscopy an attractive surgical option for animals with suspected cancer. Animals undergoing these procedures experience a short postoperative recovery and are able to be discharged to the owner while awaiting test results. With this approach, one is able to identify advanced disease that may be best treated with palliative chemotherapy on obtaining a definitive diagnosis. Because of the minimally invasive approach, chemotherapy can begin sooner than with laparotomy. Feeding tubes can be placed if necessary for enteral feeding. Frequently, staging laparoscopy is performed with the owners prepared for a decision to convert to celiotomy if warranted for resection of obstructive or locally advanced disease. If the surgeon determines that an open procedure may yield more valuable information than is obtained with laparoscopy, a decision is made to convert to a laparoscopic-assisted or open procedure.

Surgical Technique

Perform staging laparoscopy with the primary port placed at the umbilicus. Insufflate the abdomen with CO_2 to visualize the abdominal contents. As with open surgery, carefully explore the abdominal cavity. Determine the size, location, and vascularity of the internal organs. Inspect the liver and gallbladder for adhesions and focal or mass lesions. Note dilation of the biliary system by elevating the gallbladder and examine the cystic, hepatic, and common bile ducts. Visualize the stomach, spleen, omentum, and urinary bladder. Often, the lesion is readily identified and biopsies are taken. Examining the duodenum and pancreas requires rotating the animal to the left and inserting a second 5-mm port to introduce grasping forceps to lift the duodenum and expose the right lobe of the pancreas. As with open surgery, expose the right kidney, caudal vena cava, portal vein, ureter, and ovary (if present) by retracting the duodenum medially. Thorough exploration of the intestine requires inserting two 5-mm ports so that two sets of grasping forceps can be used to trace the intestine in a "hand-over-hand" manner. Inspect the intestinal surface, blood supply, and lymph nodes. Tilt the animal to the right and retract the descending colon medially to expose the left kidney, ovary, adrenal gland, and the tip of the left pancreatic lobe. Elevate the urinary bladder and examine the space between the bladder and colon to evaluate the prostate.

In human surgery, where laparoscopic techniques are well advanced, staging laparoscopy has been used extensively in patients for cancer of the esophagus, stomach, pancreas, liver and biliary system, intestinal tract, and for staging patients with suspected non-Hodgkin lymphoma when core needle biopsy is nondiagnostic. A review of the available evidence for each application in human surgery cited the safety, indications, benefits, and recommendations for future study.[5] From this review, it seems that staging laparoscopy was safe for patients with cancer; however, the role in each patient population varied with the disease state, so individual factors must be considered. When surgical resection is intended to attempt a cure, staging laparoscopy identifies those with early-stage disease by excluding evidence of malignancy from the liver or regional lymph nodes. Staging laparoscopy in people is frequently supplemented by the use of peritoneal washings and laparoscopic ultrasound. Staging laparoscopy is not usually used in patients with colon cancer because bowel resection is usually indicated to prevent or relieve bowel obstruction. It may be performed in patients with hepatic spread, if liver lobe resection is being considered.

In our experience, diagnosis of carcinomatosis by staging laparoscopy has been most rewarding. Two cases demonstrated the benefit of this approach in facilitating decision-making. One was an older basset hound with abdominal effusion and unrewarding cytology. Radiographic and ultrasound imaging failed to identify a primary mass lesion and carcinomatosis was suspected. The owners wanted a diagnosis but not aggressive surgery. Immediately on insertion of the laparoscope, omental involvement was noted, with carcinomatosis to the abdominal wall, diaphragm, and other abdominal structures. Biopsies revealed omental adenocarcinoma with carcinomatosis. The effusion was removed, and the animal was discharged from the hospital the following day to spend an additional 2 weeks with the owner before their informed decision for euthanasia. In another case, a shih tzu had previous resection of a duodenal adenocarcinoma and returned for routine oncologic monitoring 3 months postoperatively. Abdominal ultrasound revealed echogenic regions near the abdominal wall, and fine needle aspirates were not diagnostic. Laparoscopy revealed extensive adhesions from the previous surgery and evidence of tumor spread to the body wall, diaphragm, and urinary bladder (**Fig. 1**). Biopsy samples were obtained, and the animal was dismissed the day after surgery. Biopsy results revealed adenocarcinoma; the owners were able to make an informed decision for metronomic chemotherapy.

FEEDING TUBE PLACEMENT

In addition to providing a diagnosis, laparoscopy can provide an opportunity to perform palliative surgery. In human surgery, palliative procedures performed with minimally invasive surgery include gastric and biliary bypass procedures, enteric diversion, placement of hepatic infusion pumps for local chemotherapy, and radiofrequency ablation of large liver tumors.[6] Although not commonly performed, enteral feeding tube placement is a clinically relevant palliative laparoscopic procedure for animals to provide nutritional support when the stomach must be bypassed.[7] Clem and Ota performed totally laparoscopic jejunostomy feeding tube placement in eight normal dogs by introducing the feeding tube through the body wall, suturing a Witzel tunnel laparoscopically and introducing the feeding tube into the intestine. The jejunum was also sutured to the body wall. A survival study confirmed that the tubes could be placed without leakage or narrowing of the lumen.[8] This technique requires advanced suturing skills.

Laparoscopic-assisted feeding tube placement procedures are easier to perform. Rawlings, and colleagues[9] described the placement and 30-day clinical course of

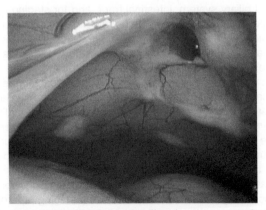

Fig. 1. Laparoscopic photograph of abdominal wall with adhesions and evidence of carcinomatosis. Biopsy samples were taken and revealed metastasis of duodenal adenocarcinoma.

laparoscopic-assisted jejunal feeding tubes in eight normal dogs. The surgical procedure involved inserting Babcock forceps through a trocar lateral to the rectus abdominis muscle to grasp the duodenum and elevate it to the body wall. The trocar was removed and the antimesenteric surface was sutured to the abdominal wall. A purse-string suture was placed in the duodenal wall, and the tube was passed through the center of the purse string and advanced into the jejunum in the same direction as intestinal contents flow. The purse-string suture was tied and a second one placed for additional reinforcement. The abdominal fascia was closed over the defect. Following this report, a comparison of laparoscopic-assisted with open surgical placement of jejunostomy tubes was performed.[10] In these procedures, the dogs were positioned in right lateral recumbency and additional time was required to determine the intestinal direction in the laparoscopic approach. A laparoscopic-assisted technique was used and eight Fr pediatric feeding tubes were placed in the jejunum. Complications were similar for the two approaches. The investigators stated that it may be easier to determine the direction of intestinal contents if the feeding tube is placed in the duodenum.[10] The dogs undergoing laparoscopic-assisted techniques were then further evaluated to compare the cardiovascular effects of general anesthesia with sedation with epidural, infusion of fentanyl-midazolam, and local anesthesia.[11] The sedation protocol proved to cause less cardiovascular depression and provided adequate analgesia for laparoscopic placement of the J-tubes. Chandler and colleagues[12] reported temporary enteric diversion on a dog with rectocutaneous fistula using a laparoscopic-assisted technique. In this case, an end-on jejunostomy was performed and, following healing of the fistula, the jejunocutaneous junction was excised and the jejunum and ileum were rejoined.[12]

Potential complications of laparoscopic-assisted feeding tube jejunostomy are the same as for open surgery. They include blockage of the feeding tube, premature dislodgement of the tube, self-mutilation, dermatitis around the ostomy site, fistula, leakage, and transient diarrhea and vomiting associated with feeding.

RETRIEVAL OF GASTRIC FOREIGN BODIES

Gastric and intestinal bezoars represent an unusual challenge in human surgery that may not be amenable to endoscopic retrieval. Thus, several investigators have performed laparoscopic retrieval in such cases.[13–15] In veterinary medicine, many gastric foreign bodies are removed using flexible endoscopy. A variety of endoscopic snares, baskets, and nets are available. If the item cannot be retrieved with an endoscopic approach and has the potential to damage the intestinal tract by remaining in place, surgery is warranted. A laparoscopic approach has been used in dogs to retrieve gastric foreign bodies.[16] In these cases, a laparoscopic approach was used to place stay sutures and to incise the stomach midway between the greater and lesser curvature. An endoscopic retrieval bag was used for removal of the foreign body, and the incision was closed with manual suturing or stapling devices. The procedure was performed in 10 dogs with various types of foreign bodies, and all recovered with no evidence of leakage and with no postoperative complications. Laparoscopic retrieval of gastric foreign bodies should be limited to those cases when the foreign body is small and compact enough to warrant a less invasive approach and when there is not a significant opportunity for spillage of gastric contents during the procedure.

GASTROPEXY

Laparoscopic-assisted gastropexy is advocated as a prophylactic procedure to prevent gastric torsion that accompanies gastric dilation in large breeds of dogs.

These procedures may be performed with laparoscopic ovariectomy or ovariohyster-ectomy in females or with castration in male dogs. Dogs with chronic gastric dilata-tion-volvulus (GDV) may also be treated with laparoscopic surgery to derotate the stomach followed by gastropexy.[17] Although other techniques for laparoscopic gas-tropexy have been advocated,[18] the laparoscopic-assisted technique described by Rawlings[19] is most widely used. The procedures are performed in large breeds of dogs 6 months and older using the following technique:

Surgical Technique

Following general anesthesia, aseptic preparation and sterile draping, begin the procedure with open insertion of a 5- or 10-mm trocar cannula approximately 3 cm caudal to the umbilicus on the ventral midline, which serves as the port for inserting the laparoscope during the procedure. Connect the laparoscope to a camera and place the monitor at the animal's head. Use a pressure-regulated CO_2 insufflator to distend the abdominal cavity and create a working space inside the abdominal cavity. Place the laparoscope in the subumbilical port for direct visualization of the next 10-mm port, which is placed approximately 3 cm caudal to the last rib just lateral to the rectus abdominis muscle on the right side of the abdomen. Next, insert 10-mm Babcock forceps to elevate the liver lobes and expose the stomach. Identify a point on the antrum of the stomach, approximately 5 cm cranial to the pylorus, for the gas-tropexy (**Fig. 2**). Use the Babcock forceps to grasp the stomach at the antrum. Move the stomach to the base of the trocar cannula and exteriorize it with the Babcock forceps by removing the cannula (**Fig. 3**). Extend the incision in the skin and abdominal fascia to 4 to 5 cm. Place two stay sutures in the gastric wall to secure the stomach, and remove the forceps. Make a seromuscular incision of the gastric wall down to, but excluding, the gastric mucosa. Suture the seromuscular layer of the stomach to the internal fascia and transverse abdominis muscle in a continuous pattern with synthetic absorbable suture. Suture the external abdominal fascia over the defect using a contin-uous pattern with synthetic absorbable suture. Insufflate the abdomen and examine the gastropexy site laparoscopically to ensure no twisting of the stomach occurred (**Fig. 4**). Administer postoperative analgesics and discharge the dog the following day with instructions for limited activity for 10 to 14 days. The most common post-operative complication from this procedure is seroma formation at the incision site, which can usually be managed conservatively.

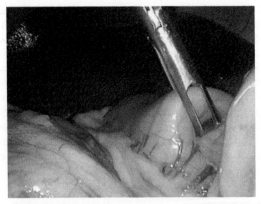

Fig. 2. Laparoscopic view of Babcock forceps grasping the stomach wall midway between the greater and lesser curvatures about 5 cm proximal to the pylorus.

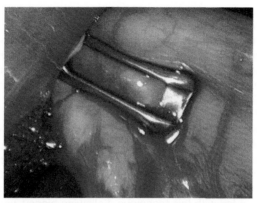

Fig. 3. Laparoscopic view taken after the 10-mm trocar was withdrawn, showing the Babcock forceps bringing the stomach to the body wall. This photograph was taken while stay sutures were being applied from outside the body.

In the past, several investigators have studied the tensile strength of the gastropexy;[18,20] however, it is not known how strong the adhesion has to be to prevent rotation of the distended stomach. Rawlings demonstrated tensile strength of the gastropexy sites in laparoscopic-assisted technique equivalent to other methods in his original technique description.[19] He followed 20 dogs 1 year following surgery with ultrasound imaging and showed persistence of the adhesions at the gastropexy site in those animals.[17]

INTESTINAL BIOPSY

Laparoscopic biopsy of the stomach and intestines is a minimally invasive method for obtaining full-thickness biopsy samples necessary to make accurate diagnoses. Evans and colleagues[21] compared the diagnostic accuracy of mucosal biopsy samples obtained with endoscopic technique to full-thickness biopsy samples obtained with surgery in cats with inflammatory bowel disease or lymphosarcoma. In this study, lymphosarcoma was diagnosed in 10 cats on the basis of full-thickness biopsy. In the stomach, full-thickness biopsy diagnosed lymphosarcoma in 4 cats,

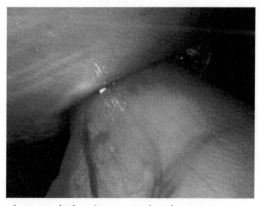

Fig. 4. Laparoscopic photograph showing a completed gastropexy.

compared with 3 cats undergoing endoscopic biopsy. However, in the intestine, full-thickness biopsy detected lymphosarcoma in the jejunum and ileum in 10 cats and in the duodenum in 9 cats, whereas 4 incorrect diagnoses of inflammatory bowel disease were made with endoscopic biopsy in cats that actually had lymphosarcoma.[21] There were no complications from the surgical procedures. Laparoscopic-assisted intestinal biopsy is simple to perform and yields valuable information for decision-making.

Surgical Technique

Following an exploratory laparoscopy, remove the primary port and extend the umbilical incision cranially and caudally on midline for approximately 5 cm. Grasp a loop of intestine and exteriorize and trace it cranially to the stomach and caudally to the colon. Pack off the incision with moistened laparotomy pads, obtain full-thickness samples of the intestine, and close the incision with routine suturing (**Fig. 5**). Enlarged lymph nodes can also be sampled with this technique. Following biopsy, wrap the intestine in omentum and replace it in the abdominal cavity. If necessary, resection and anastomosis can be performed instead of biopsy using traditional suturing techniques. Close the body wall, subcutaneous tissue, and skin routinely. If desired during closure, reinsert the camera port, and following insufflation, inspect and lavage the abdomen. Following postoperative recovery, give the animal analgesics and offer water at 6 hours, with feeding beginning at 12 hours postoperatively.

LAPAROSCOPIC ORGAN BIOPSY

Laparoscopic organ biopsy is one of the simplest minimally invasive procedures to perform and is frequently requested in our hospital. After considering other less invasive and less costly means to obtain tissue, such as ultrasound-guided fine needle aspirates or percutaneous biopsy, internists request laparoscopy biopsy because they desire visual examination of the abdominal organs, and because they need multiple biopsies or larger tissue samples than are obtained by less invasive methods. They also may want visual confirmation of hemostasis, or they may desire ancillary procedures such as gallbladder aspirates for culture/sensitivity. The most

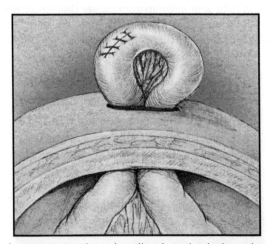

Fig. 5. The umbilical trocar site is enlarged to allow bowel to be brought externally. A biopsy or intestinal anastomosis may be performed. (*From* Freeman LJ, editor. Veterinary endosurgery. Mosby: St Louis (MO); 1999. p. 136; with permission.)

commonly performed solid organ biopsy procedures involve obtaining tissue specimens from the liver, kidney, spleen, pancreas, and lymph nodes. The following techniques are used to obtain samples for biopsy:

Surgical Technique

Following general anesthesia, if systemic disease is suspected, place the animal in left lateral recumbency for liver biopsy, as approximately 85% of the liver can be visualized and the procedure is technically simpler. If focal disease is present on ultrasound examination, or if there are other abdominal abnormalities, the animal is positioned in dorsal recumbence to enable visualization of each of the liver lobes and a thorough exploration of the abdomen. The surgical site is prepared and draped accordingly.

Make a 5- to 7-mm incision through the skin with a no. 15 scalpel blade. For animals positioned in dorsal recumbency, place the initial port just caudal to the umbilicus, avoiding the umbilical fat pad. If the animal is positioned in lateral recumbency, place the primary port at a point halfway between the caudal border of the ribs and the wing of the ilium and midway between the spine and ventral midline. Excise the underlying subcutaneous tissue with Metzenbaum scissors down to the abdominal fascia. Elevate the fascia and make a small incision through the fascia, abdominal musculature, and peritoneum. To prevent loss of pneumoperitoneum during the procedure, the incision in the fascia should be no larger than the diameter of the trocar shaft. Confirm entry into the abdominal cavity and place two stay sutures through the abdominal fascia to secure the fascia to the trocar. These sutures can be tied around the stopcock, or around an olive plug positioned on the trocar cannula. Following insufflation and visualization, place secondary ports for biopsy.

Carefully introduce each instrument into the abdominal cavity under direct visualization to avoid injury to underlying structures. For hemostasis, place absorbable golatin compressed sponge (Gelfoam Sponge, Pfizer Inc., New York, New York) inside the abdomen before obtaining biopsy samples. To introduce the Gelfoam, use an introducer sleeve and plastic push rod from a pretied loop ligature system (SURGITIE single use ligating loop with delivery system; Covidien, Mansfield, Massachusetts). Break three or four pieces of dry Gelfoam off the sheet, roll them into 3- to 4-mm cylinders, and back-load them into the introducer cannula (**Fig. 6**). Insert the cannula into the working port and push the Gelfoam samples into the abdominal cavity with the plastic push rod (**Fig. 7**). Ideally, position the samples near where the biopsy samples

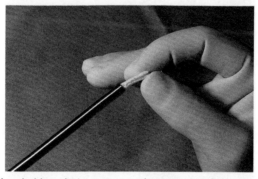

Fig. 6. A piece of absorbable gelatin compressed sponge is rolled up and inserted into an introducer sleeve from a pretied loop ligature system (Surgitie, Covidien, Mansfield, Massachusetts). The introducer sleeve makes it easier to introduce the sponge into the trocar.

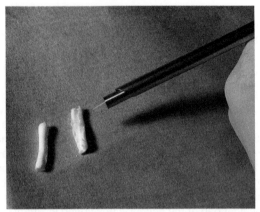

Fig. 7. The plastic push rod is used to push the pieces of sponge into the abdominal cavity.

are to be taken (**Figs. 8–10**). After obtaining the sample, place the Gelfoam in the defect, and apply pressure for approximately 1 minute.

Biopsy Cup Forceps

Use laparoscopic biopsy cup forceps to obtain tissue specimens from any solid organ with minimal hemorrhage. Insert the forceps, position them on tissue, and close them. Maintain the forceps in position for approximately 30 seconds, close them more tightly, then twist and pull to retrieve the sample (**Fig. 11**). Remove the forceps, place the sample in a saline-moistened gauze sponge, and pass it off the surgical field. Introduce grasping forceps to "nudge" the Gelfoam samples into the tissue defect (**Fig. 12**).

Loop Ligature Technique

A pretied loop ligature (Endoloop, Ethicon, Inc, Somerville, New Jersey) can be a useful tool in ensuring hemostasis following biopsy of the pancreas. Endoloop application requires a minimum of two ports in addition to the camera port. Use one for introducing the Endoloop and the other for a grasping forceps. Introduce the Endoloop

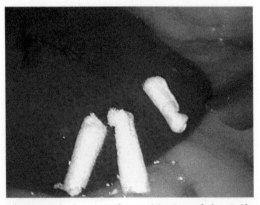

Fig. 8. Laparoscopic photograph showing the positioning of the Gelfoam pledgets before obtaining a biopsy of a liver mass.

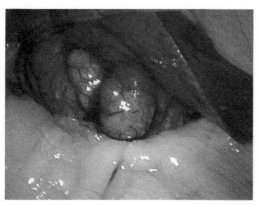

Fig. 9. Laparoscopic photograph of a liver mass in a 16-year-old cat. The mass was diagnosed as hepatocellular carcinoma following biopsy.

into the trocar, taking care to avoid the flapper valve mechanism. Once inside the body cavity, bring the grasping forceps through the loop and to the tissue to be removed (**Fig. 13**). Grasp the tissue and elevate it with the Endoloop positioned around the tissue to be removed. Position the tip of the pusher cannula at the site of desired knot placement. After the loop is tightened, use laparoscopic scissors to excise and remove the tissue specimen. Cut the suture approximately 2 mm from the knot.

Needle Biopsy

The Tru-Cut biopsy needle (Allegiance Health Care Corporation, McGaw Park, Illinois) is most often used to obtain samples of the renal cortex, but may also be used to obtain samples of the liver, spleen, or lymph node. Renal biopsy is performed to evaluate renal masses and suspected glomerular diseases to enable the clinician to formulate specific treatment recommendations and determine short- and long-term prognosis. Pathologists use criteria established by human renopathologists to thoroughly evaluate renal biopsies and establish diagnoses. The surgeon must provide a sample that includes a minimum number of intact glomeruli, renal arterioles, and

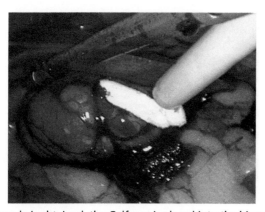

Fig. 10. After the sample is obtained, the Gelfoam is placed into the biopsy defect and pressure is applied.

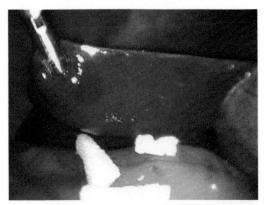

Fig. 11. Five millimeter cup biopsy forceps are positioned on a focal liver lesion. Pressure is applied for approximately 30 seconds and the forceps are twisted and pulled to remove the tissue.

cortical interstitium. Most renal biopsies are obtained percutaneously under ultrasound guidance using spring-loaded biopsy needles. Two to three biopsies are usually required to provide sufficient tissue for evaluation by light, immunofluorescence, and electron microscopy. Unfortunately, each needle pass increases the risk of complications. To obtain larger samples and enable observation of post biopsy bleeding, the following laparoscopic techniques are frequently used:

Surgical Technique

In this procedure, a minimum of two ports are required, one for the laparoscope and one for a grasping forceps. If both kidneys require biopsy, the ideal location for port placement is the ventral midline. Position the animal in lateral recumbency with the affected kidney up. Stabilize the kidney with a grasping forceps and introduce the needle percutaneously at an angle directed away from the hilus. During renal biopsy, the goal is to obtain a minimum of 10 glomeruli for histologic examination, and more is better.[22] Depending on the needle size, multiple samples are taken. During a laparoscopic teaching laboratory, participants took samples with a 14-gauge biopsy device.

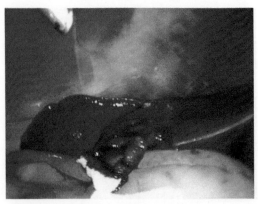

Fig. 12. Several liver biopsy samples are taken for culture, pathology, impression cytology, and metal analysis. The Gelfoam is placed in the defect to assist with hemostasis.

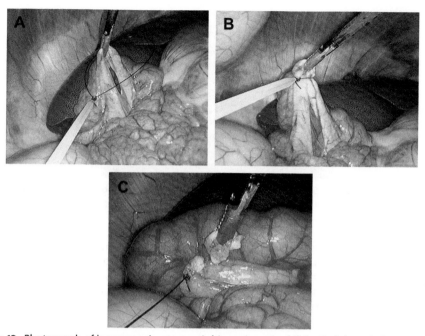

Fig. 13. Photograph of laparoscopic pancreatic biopsy in a pig. (*A*) An Endoloop (Ethicon, Inc, Somerville, New Jersey) is used to snare a portion of the pancreas that is being elevated by the grasping forceps. (*From* Freeman LJ, editor. Veterinary endosurgery. St. Louis (MO): Mosby; 1999. Plate 18; with permission.) (*B*) The loop is tightened by advancing the plastic push rod. (*From* Freeman LJ, editor. Veterinary endosurgery. St. Louis (MO): Mosby; 1999. Plate 19; with permission). (*C*) The tissue is cut free and removed. (*From* Freeman LJ, editor. Veterinary endosurgery. St. Louis (MO): Mosby; 1999. Plate 20; with permission.)

These laparoscopically viewed renal biopsy procedures resulted in high-quality specimens with an adequate number of glomeruli for evaluation.[23] Following biopsy, hemorrhage from the biopsy site is usually managed by pressure and Gelfoam application.

The author has had difficulty in obtaining diagnostic renal biopsy samples using traditional 16-gauge needles and is exploring a new vacuum-assisted biopsy device (Celero, Hologic, Inc., Indianapolis, Indiana) (**Fig. 14**). The Celero device is a 12-gauge biopsy device designed for ultrasound-guided biopsy of the human breast. Similar to other spring-loaded devices, the obturator/sample chamber advances slightly ahead of the cutting obturator. Unique to the Celero design, vacuum is applied to the tissue (similar to aspirating a syringe) to bring the sample into the chamber before the cutting obturator severs the sample from the surrounding tissue. The device is then removed, the outer cannula retracted to expose the specimen chamber, and the sample is removed. Preliminary studies indicate that the device obtains high-quality samples with moderate intraoperative bleeding that is controlled by application of pressure and Gelfoam.

Renal hemorrhage is the most commonly reported complication following renal biopsy, which may result in perirenal or renal hematomas, hematuria, arteriovenous fistula formation, and hydronephrosis if the ureter becomes obstructed by a clot. These complications are most likely associated with inadvertent biopsy of a larger renal arcuate artery or other vessels; other complications that may result from

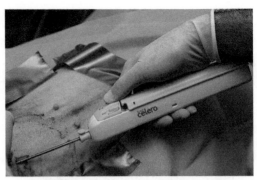

Fig. 14. Photograph of Suros Celero a 12-gauge vacuum-assisted biopsy device made by Hologic, Inc. (Indianapolis, Indiana) being used to obtain tissue biopsy samples in a female dog.

compromise of the renal vasculature during biopsy include infarction, thrombosis, significant decrease in renal function, and in some cases death.[24] The complication rate, including life-threatening sequela and minor findings such as hematuria, is 13.4% in dogs. Severe hemorrhage occurred in 9.9% of dogs and death in 2.5% of dogs in the largest veterinary study reported.[25]

Excisional Biopsy

Laparoscopic excisional biopsy is most often performed for evaluation of lymph nodes. Enlarged lymph nodes may be classified as reactive, be involved with a primary disease process such as lymphosarcoma, or be involved as a site of metastasis of primary neoplasia. The sentinel lymph node is the first node or group of nodes in a lymphatic pattern draining a site. Therefore, they are the most likely to contain cancer cells that metastasize from a primary tumor. In human surgery, mapping of the sentinel lymph node is performed by injecting blue dye or radioactive substances near the primary lesion and observing its spread to regional lymph nodes. The sentinel node or nodes are removed and if they are negative, the patient is spared more radical surgery. In human surgery, laparoscopic evaluation of sentinel lymph nodes has been reported for staging patients with gastric, colonic, cervical, uterine, and prostate cancer. Usually, radioactive isotopes and a hand-held gamma probe are used to identify the affected node.

In veterinary medicine, affected lymph nodes are more commonly identified by size or location adjacent to a region of interest. In these cases, the lymph nodes are visualized laparoscopically and carefully dissected from the surrounding tissue. The harmonic scalpel can be a helpful dissection tool (**Figs. 15** and **16**).

Fine Needle Aspirate

A fine needle aspirate can be performed in any organ under laparoscopic visualization. The authors frequently perform gallbladder aspirates to obtain samples of bile for culture; however, the technique can also be used for other cystic or solid structures.

Surgical Technique

In this procedure, stabilize the gallbladder with a grasping forceps and insert a 2.5-inch spinal needle percutaneously. Take care to avoid penetration of the diaphragm, which could result in tension pneumothorax when the abdominal cavity is insufflated. After the needle penetrates the gallbladder, remove the stylet and attach the syringe to

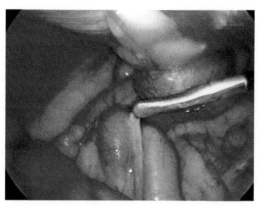

Fig. 15. Laparoscopic image of an enlarged colonic lymph node in a 10-year-old cat.

obtain a fluid sample. When sufficient fluid is removed to obtain samples for analysis and to slightly decompress the gallbladder, withdraw the needle. Keep the needle entry point in direct vision to ensure cessation of leakage. If necessary, reposition the forceps to close the hole in the gallbladder.

Final Inspection

Final inspection of the abdominal cavity is performed to ensure hemostasis before closure. If there is concern for active bleeding, it may be necessary to irrigate the site or lavage the abdomen and aspirate the fluid. If the animal is hypotensive during surgery, when the abdominal pressure is reduced and the blood pressure returns to normal, bleeding can occur. Each of the ancillary trocars are removed, and the incisions in the fascia, subcutaneous tissue, and skin are closed with small sutures.

Most animals undergoing laparoscopic organ biopsy are ill and return to the intensive care unit for recovery and follow up care. Simple cases are sent home on the day of surgery, and the owners are called the following morning. Postoperative care includes monitoring for signs of pain, bleeding, and hypoglycemia. Medical management is continued until a definitive diagnosis is obtained.

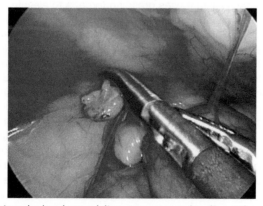

Fig. 16. The harmonic scalpel and curved dissector were used to dissect the node and remove it.

LAPAROSCOPIC COLON RESECTION

Laparoscopic resection of the intestine is frequently performed in people, but rarely in animals. Potential reasons are the small body cavity, the high cost of stapling equipment, and the lack of experience with laparoscopic techniques. For these reasons, it will likely remain much simpler and faster to perform a laparoscopic-assisted procedure if intestinal resection is necessary in animals.[26,27] Laparoscopic colon resection and anastomosis was performed in a 10-year-old female Labrador retriever using the following technique.

Careful case selection is critical for satisfactory outcomes. A benign or locally invasive tumor involving the distal colon above the pelvic inlet is the ideal candidate. For optimal presurgical bowel preparation, the mass should not be obstructive. Fast the animal, perform oral gavage with PEG-350 and Electrolytes for Oral Solution (Go-Lytely; Braintree Laboratories, Inc, Braintree, Massachusetts) and administer presurgical cleansing enemas beginning 24 hours before surgery. Express the bladder before surgery and administer perioperative antimicrobials. Presurgical planning is necessary to ensure that (1) the mass can be identified with laparoscopic visualization, (2) a minimum of 1-cm margins of normal tissue are available proximal and distal to the lesion, and (3) the lesion can be resected without unacceptable tension on the surgical anastomosis. Special instruments needed during the procedure include a circular stapler having an outer diameter that allows it to be inserted through the pelvic canal (usually 21 or 25 mm) and an endoscopic linear stapler that is capable of being reloaded. A disposable purse-string device, large (18 or 33 mm) trocar and a laparoscopic anvil grasper are helpful, but not absolutely necessary. In addition, a sigmoidoscope may be necessary for final examination of the staple line.

Surgical Technique

Following general anesthesia, position the animal with the anus at the end of the surgical table to facilitate future introduction of a surgical stapler. Place the monitor at the foot of the table. Clip and prepare the abdomen for aseptic surgery and drape to enable celiotomy, if necessary. Use an open technique to place a Hasson trocar at the umbilicus to serve as the camera port. After insufflation to 12 mmHg, perform a visual exploratory of the abdominal cavity and take samples of the liver for staging purposes. Place 5-mm ports in the right and left cranial abdominal quadrants. Place a 10-mm port in the caudal right quadrant. Tilt the head down to expose the descending colon. The surgical assistant uses grasping forceps to elevate the colon and the lesion is identified. Remove the colonic lymph node in the region for staging. Dissect the short colonic vessels (**Fig. 17**) and ligate with clips or coagulate and cut them with a harmonic scalpel, preserving the blood supply to the distal colon. Continue the dissection a minimum of 1 cm proximal and distal to the lesion, ideally obtaining 2-cm margins. Introduce an endoscopic linear stapler, such as the EndoGIA 60, through the 10-mm port and use it to transect the colon distal to the lesion. Exteriorize the proximal portion of colon by removing the trocar and enlarge the caudal right quadrant port to accept the anvil of the circular stapler. Clamp the colon proximal to the lesion to prevent spillage of intestinal contents and transect proximal to the lesion. Submit the specimen for histopathologic examination. Place a purse-string suture of 2-0 Prolene around the proximal portion of bowel. Separate the anvil of the circular stapler, introduce it into the proximal bowel, and tighten the purse-string suture around the anvil post. Replace the proximal bowel containing the anvil into the abdominal cavity (**Fig. 18**).

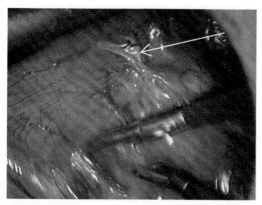

Fig. 17. The blood supply to the descending colon is provided by the caudal mesenteric artery, which follows the border of the descending colon, giving off numerous short branches (vasa recta) to supply the colon. It becomes the left colic artery proximally and the cranial rectal artery distally. Dissection is performed in the thin mesentery between the vessel and the colon. A colonic mass is suspected by the abnormal vasculature on the surface of the colon (*white arrow*).

Reestablish pneumoperitoneum by closing the incision or by placing a large trocar to prevent loss of insufflation. Introduce the other end of the circular stapler transanally and advance it to the staple line. Visualize the flat end of the stapler adjacent to or overlapping the linear staple line. Extend the trocar of the circular stapler until the visual tab is seen. Place and secure the anvil post extending from the proximal bowel over the trocar. Examine the mesentery to ensure that it is aligned and there is no twisting. Close and fire the circular stapler to perform the anastomosis (**Fig. 19**).

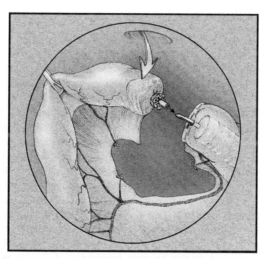

Fig. 18. A purse-string suture is placed around the anvil shaft in the proximal portion of bowel. The stapler is introduced through the rectum and the trocar tip is extended just beside the distal staple line. The anvil shaft is joined with the trocar from the circular stapler. (*From* Freeman LJ, editor. Veterinary endosurgery. St. Louis (MO): Mosby; 1999. p. 148; with permission.)

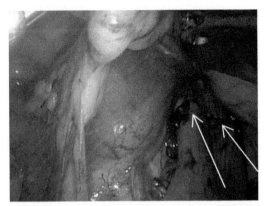

Fig. 19. Laparoscopic photograph of the completed colonic anastomosis (*arrows*).

Remove the stapler and examine the tissue donuts to ensure complete anastomosis, and submit the sample for histopathologic examination. Usually it is not necessary to close the colonic mesentery to prevent internal herniation. Perform a thorough lavage of the abdominal cavity and close the trocar sites routinely.

Postoperative care is the same as for animals undergoing open celiotomy, with postoperative analgesia, nutritional support and gradual introduction of feeding, and oral antibiotic therapy. Monitor the animal for evidence of postoperative leakage and discontinue monitoring when intestinal motility is evident without sepsis. The procedure was successfully accomplished, and the diagnosis was colonic carcinoma. The lymph node was reactive, but did not contain neoplastic cells. Five days following surgery, the dog developed a wound infection in the large trocar site, which was managed conservatively with antibiotics and has recovered uneventfully.

LAPAROSCOPIC CHOLECYSTECTOMY

Laparoscopic cholecystectomy has become the standard of care for treatment of gall-bladder disease resulting from cholelithiasis in man but has not been adopted in veterinary medicine. Cholecystectomy is rarely performed in animals and is usually a result of cholecystitis that does not respond to medical management, gallbladder mucocele, neoplasia, or rupture. In these cases, the gallbladder is distended, friable, and may be difficult to manipulate without iatrogenic rupture. In small animals, the optical cavity may be limited, making a laparoscopic approach more challenging. Yet, there may be advantages of the laparoscopic approach versus open surgery when it can be performed safely. Studies comparing open with laparoscopic cholecystectomy in dogs have shown less extensive adhesions following laparoscopic procedures.[28] The investigators concluded from this study that because of higher white blood cell counts in peritoneal lavage specimens, the laparosopic approach was associated with an improved cell-mediated response and therefore less suppression of the immune response. Other investigators studying gastrointestinal motility in dogs following open and laparoscopic cholecystectomy concluded that more rapid gastric emptying following feeding was seen in the animals undergoing laparoscopic procedures.[29] Mayhew and colleagues[30] reported performing laparoscopic cholecystectomy in 6 dogs with gallbladder mucoceles. In the Mayhew study, case selection was limited to animals with uncomplicated disease. Animals with gallbladder rupture or those with evidence of extrahepatic biliary tract obstruction were excluded from the laparosopic approach. The surgical technique follows. For additional information, see the article on laparoscopic cholecystectomy in this issue.

Surgical Technique

With the monitor positioned at the head of the table and following primary port placement for the laparoscope and insufflation of the abdominal cavity, place three additional working ports, two located to the right of the umbilicus and one to the left. Place a fan retractor in the left port and pass it under the falciform ligament to expose the cystic duct. A working knowledge of the anatomy of the canine cystic duct and common bile duct is essential to avoid inadvertent ligation of the common bile duct. Use right-angled forceps to dissect the cystic duct and artery. A combination of endoscopic ligating clips and extracorporeally tied sutures are used to ligate the cystic duct and artery, with care taken to ensure that the suture remaining on the gallbladder is securely placed and gently manipulated to avoid spilling bile during the procedure. Elevate the neck of the gallbladder and dissect the gallbladder from the liver with a hook electrocautery or ultracision device. When the dissection is complete, place the gallbladder in a specimen retrieval bag for removal from the umbilicus. Lavage the abdomen with saline and close the port sites routinely. Following surgery, administer fluids, antibiotics, analgesics, and NSAIDs and feed a normal diet the day after surgery.

Laparoscopic cholecystectomy is considered the gold standard operation for human patients for treatment of cholelithiasis. However, when surgeons first began to perform these operations, there were several complications, including iatrogenic injury. Vessel injuries from Veress needle or trocar placement occurred. There was damage to the intestine, bile leakage, spilling gallstones in the patient, and the most serious injury involved accidental ligation of the common bile duct. In addition, bleeding from the cystic artery and gallbladder bed were also noted. Today, the complication rate for laparoscopic cholecystectomy in people is less than 2% and most can be managed conservatively if recognized early.[31] As veterinarians are beginning to perform more complicated procedures, the wise surgeon will select cases carefully, recognize the potential for significant complications, and be willing to convert to an open procedure if it becomes necessary.

FUTURE DIRECTION

In human medicine, there is movement toward "scarless" surgery for procedures in the abdominal cavity. One approach involves entering the body through a natural orifice and performing entire procedures with a two-channel flexible endoscope with access through the stomach, colon, vagina, or bladder. This approach is known as natural orifice translumenal endoscopic surgery (NOTES). The modern day approach was first reported by Dr. Anthony Kalloo of Johns Hopkins University in 2004.[32] He and his colleagues used a system of guide wires, an endoscopic needle knife, and balloon dilators to gain access to the abdominal cavity through the gastric wall with a flexible endoscope in pigs. Room air from the endoscope was used to insufflate the abdominal cavity and he called the technique "peritoneoscopy." Since that time, several experimental procedures have been performed in animals and human cholecystectomies have been performed using the gastric and vaginal access routes. Hybrid procedures are being performed using flexible endoscopy and traditional laparoscopic instruments inserted through an umbilical port. Instrument manufacturers are currently working to develop instruments specific for this application as the application of this technology is being expanded to other procedural areas. There are still several unanswered questions regarding the new technique. The best method of preparing the organ for sterile surgery is unknown. Long-term outcomes are unknown. To date, researchers have not demonstrated conclusive evidence that the NOTES procedures are indeed less invasive. Nevertheless, there is a great deal of interest in these procedures and there are more than 50 groups around the world working to evaluate and develop these techniques for human surgery.

Another attempt to reduce the invasiveness of minimally invasive surgery is by placing only one port at the umbilicus. Several approaches, single incision laparoscopic surgery (SILS), single port access surgery, and one port umbilical surgery (OPUS) have evolved. Currently, the term laparoendoscopic single site surgery (LESS) is the preferred term.[33] In this procedure, several devices are inserted through either one large port that has multiple channels, or through small adjacent trocars. Using a combination of a rigid endoscope that has a flexible tip and instruments that articulate, surgeons are able to achieve triangulation at an operative site. These techniques and procedures are in an early stage of development and it is unknown at this time whether they will be proven equivalent to or better than traditional laparoscopy.

SUMMARY

Although adoption of minimally invasive surgery in veterinary medicine lags behind human surgery in many areas, laparoscopic procedures that involve the gastrointestinal tract are feasible and can be performed safely in animals. Veterinarians wishing to extend the practice of minimally invasive surgery should consider laparoscopic-assisted techniques as viable alternatives to total laparoscopic procedures, as they offer benefits of reduced incision size and rapid recovery from surgery. Growth of minimally invasive procedures in veterinary medicine is anticipated as technology continues to advance, clients demand better care for their pets, and as surgeons gain familiarity with new techniques.

REFERENCES

1. MacPhail CM, Monnet E, Twedt DC. Thoracoscopic correction of persistent right aortic arch in a dog. J Am Anim Hosp Assoc 2001;37:577–81.
2. Koontz CS, Bhatia A, Forbess J, et al. Video-assisted thoracoscopic division of vascular rings in pediatric patients. Am Surg 2005;71(4):289–91.
3. Suematsu Y, Mora BN, Mihaljevic T, et al. Totally endoscopic robotic-assisted repair of patent ductus arteriosus and vascular ring in children. Ann Thorac Surg 2005;80(6):2309–13.
4. Kogon BE, Forbess JM, Wulkan ML, et al. Video-assisted thoracoscopic surgery: is it a superior technique for the division of vascular rings in children? Congenit Heart Dis 2007;2(2):130–3.
5. Chang L, Stefanidis D, Richardson WS, et al. The role of staging laparoscopy for intraabdominal cancers: an evidence-based review. Surg Endosc 2009;23(2): 231–41.
6. Torab FC, Bokobza B, Branicki F. Laparoscopy in gastrointestinal malignancies. Ann N Y Acad Sci 2008;1138:155–61.
7. Cavanaugh RP, Kovak JR, Fischetti AJ, et al. Evaluation of surgically placed gastrojejunostomy feeding tubes in critically ill dogs. J Am Vet Med Assoc 2008;232: 380–8.
8. Freeman LJ. Minimally invasive small intestinal surgery. In: Freeman LJ, editor. Veterinary endosurgery. St Louis (MO): Mosby; 1999. p. 133–43.

9. Rawlings CA, Howerth EW, Bement S, et al. Laparoscopic-assisted enterostomy tube placement and full-thickness biopsy of the jejunum with serosal patching in dogs. Am J Vet Res 2002;63(9):1313–9.
10. Hewitt SA, Brisson BA, Sinclair MD, et al. Evaluation of laparoscopic-assisted placement of jejunostomy feeding tubes in dogs. J Am Vet Med Assoc 2004; 225(1):65–71.
11. Hewitt SA, Brisson BA, Sinclair MD, et al. Comparison of cardiopulmonary responses during sedation with epidural and local anesthesia for laparo-scopic-assisted jejunostomy feeding tube placement with cardiopulmonary responses during general anesthesia for laparoscopic-assisted or open surgical jejunostomy feeding tube placement in healthy dogs. Am J Vet Res 2007;68(4): 358–69.
12. Chandler JC, Kudnig ST, Monnet E. Use of laparoscopic-assisted jejunostomy for fecal diversion in the management of a rectocutaneous fistula in a dog. J Am Vet Med Assoc 2005;226(5):746–51.
13. Song KY, Choi BJ, Kim SN, et al. Laparoscopic removal of gastric bezoar. Surg Laparosc Endosc Percutan Tech 2007;17(1):42–4.
14. Shami SB, Jararaa AA, Hamade A, et al. Laparoscopic removal of a huge gastric trichobezoar in a patient with trichotillomania. Surg Laparosc Endosc Percutan Tech 2007;17(3):197–200.
15. Nirasawa Y, Mori T, Ito Y, et al. Laparoscopic removal of a large gastric trichobe-zoar. J Pediatr Surg 1998;33(4):663–5.
16. Lew M, Jałynski M, Brzeski W. Laparoscopic removal of gastric foreign bodies in dogs – comparison of manual suturing and stapling viscerosynthesis. Pol J Vet Sci 2005;8(2):147–53.
17. Rawlings CA, Mahaffey MB, Bement S, et al. Prospective evaluation of laparo-scopic-assisted gastropexy in dogs susceptible to gastric dilatation. J Am Vet Med Assoc 2002;221(11):1576–81.
18. Hardie RJ, Flanders JA, Schmidt P, et al. Biomechanical and histological evalua-tion of a laparoscopic stapled gastropexy technique in dogs. Vet Surg 1996; 25(2):127–33.
19. Rawlings CA, Foutz TL, Mahaffey MB, et al. A rapid and strong laparoscopic-as-sisted gastropexy in dogs. Am J Vet Res 2001;62(6):871–5.
20. Wilson ER, Henderson RA, Montgomery RD, et al. A comparison of laparoscopic and belt-loop gastropexy in dogs. Vet Surg 1996;25(3):221–7.
21. Evans SE, Bonczynski JJ, Broussard JD, et al. Comparison of endoscopic and full-thickness biopsy specimens for diagnosis of inflammatory bowel disease and alimentary tract lymphoma in cats. J Am Vet Med Assoc 2006;229(9): 1447–50.
22. Corwin HL, Schwartz MM, Lewis EJ. The importance of sample size in the inter-pretation of the renal biopsy. Am J Nephrol 1988;8(2):85–9.
23. Rawlings CA, Diamond H, Howerth EW, et al. Diagnostic quality of percutaneous kidney biopsy specimens obtained with laparoscopy versus ultrasound guidance in dogs. J Am Vet Med Assoc 2003;223(3):317–21.
24. Vaden SL. Renal biopsy: methods and interpretation. Vet Clin North Am Small Anim Pract 2004;34:887–908.
25. Vaden SL, Levine JF, Lees GE, et al. Renal biopsy: a retrospective study of methods and complications in 283 dogs and 65 cats. J Vet Intern Med 2005; 19(6):794–801.
26. Davies W, Kollmorgen CF, Tu QM, et al. Laparoscopic colectomy shortens post-operative ileus in a canine model. Surgery 1997;121(5):550–5.

27. Tittel A, Schippers E, Anurov M, et al. Shorter postoperative atony after laparo-scopic-assisted colonic resection? An animal study. Surg Endosc 2001;15(5): 508–12.

28. Szabó G, Mikó I, Nagy P, et al. Adhesion formation with open versus laparoscopic cholecystectomy: an immunologic and histologic study. Surg Endosc 2007;21(2): 253–7.

29. Hotokezaka M, Combs MJ, Mentis EP, et al. Recovery of fasted and fed gastro-intestinal motility after open versus laparoscopic cholecystectomy in dogs. Ann Surg 1996;223(4):413–9.

30. Mayhew PD, Mehler SJ, Radhakrishnan A. Laparoscopic cholecystectomy for management of uncomplicated gall bladder mucocele in six dogs. Vet Surg 2008;37(7):625–30.

31. Shamiyeh A, Wayand W. Laparoscopic cholecystectomy: early and late compli-cations and their treatment. Langenbecks Arch Surg 2004;389:164–71.

32. Kalloo AN, Singh VK, Jagannath SB, et al. Flexible transgastric peritoneoscopy: a novel approach to diagnostic and therapeutic interventions in the peritoneal cavity. Gastrointest Endosc 2004;60(1):114–7.

33. Box G, Averch T, Cadeddu J, et al. Nomenclature of natural orifice translumenal endoscopic surgery (NOTES) and laparoendoscopic single-site surgery (LESS) procedures in urology. J Endourol 2008;22(11):2575–81.

Advanced Laparoscopic Procedures (Hepatobiliary, Endocrine) in Dogs and Cats

Philipp D. Mayhew, BVM&S, MRCVS

KEYWORDS

- Laparoscopy • Adrenalectomy • Cholecystectomy
- Minimally invasive • Mucocele

As laparoscopic procedures become more popular in veterinary medicine and surgeons' experience increases, there is a natural trend toward the development of more complex interventions. The list of procedures that can now be performed laparoscopically is growing rapidly. Many advanced laparoscopic procedures were first performed in human medicine in the late 1980s and early 1990s, including cholecystectomy and adrenalectomy. Cholecystectomy lent itself so well to a laparoscopic approach that this has become the procedure of choice for management of cholelithiasis and acute cholecystitis in humans; more than 75% of cholecystectomies in North America are performed laparoscopically.[1] This procedure has evolved further in humans to include adjunctive interventions such as intraoperative cholangiography and laparoscopic common bile duct exploration.[2] This evolution in human medicine is likely to be mirrored in veterinary medicine, although care must be taken to ensure that the same standards of care expected for "open" procedures are upheld for minimally invasive interventions.

Cholecystectomy and adrenalectomy have now been described in veterinary patients for management of select cases.[3,4] With all advanced interventions, several factors are important for achieving success: strict case selection, possession of the equipment necessary to perform the procedure safely and efficiently, and proper advanced training. Without these factors little success can be expected, and conversions to an open approach will be commonplace. The surgeon should remember, however, that safety is paramount, and a liberal policy of conversion to an open approach should not be viewed as failure but as evidence of good surgical judgment.

Columbia River Veterinary Specialists, 6818 NE Fourth Plain Boulevard, Vancouver, WA 98661, USA

E-mail address: philmayhew@gmail.com

Vet Clin Small Anim 39 (2009) 925–939
doi:10.1016/j.cvsm.2009.05.004
0195-5616/09/$ – see front matter
vetsmall.theclinics.com

Owners should always be made aware of the risk of conversion, and the clinician should not proceed if there is an unwillingness to convert to an open approach.

The advantage of completing these procedures laparoscopically has been well researched in human medicine; it is known that laparoscopic cholecystectomy results in decreased postoperative pain, more rapid return to normal activity, and improved cosmesis.[5] Newer evidence is emerging of other significant advantages to minimally invasive approaches. One study comparing open and laparoscopic adrenalectomy showed that the laparoscopic group experienced fewer postoperative complications such as pneumonia, sepsis, and wound infections.[6] Some studies in small animals have shown reduced pain[7,8] and a more rapid return to normal activity[9,10] after laparoscopic surgery. Future studies will likely evaluate whether some of the other morbidities mentioned are reduced when minimally invasive procedures are used in place of open surgery in dogs and cats.

INSTRUMENTATION

An endoscopic tower is necessary to perform any laparoscopic interventions. The tower contains a video monitor, a camera, a light source with light cable, a mechanical insufflator, and a recording device (either a printer or a digital image recording device). A laparoscope is used to transmit the images back to the camera. The laparoscope is usually 5 or 10 mm in diameter and has a viewing angle of either 0° or 30°. The 5-mm laparoscope offers an ideal balance between adequate light transmission for visualization of relevant anatomy in medium to large dogs while maintaining small port incisions. The 30° viewing angle allows for a greater field of view when the laparoscope is rotated, but it is more difficult for inexperienced laparoscopists to manipulate. For the procedures discussed in this article, a 0° or 30° laparoscope can used interchangeably.

Three to four trocar-cannula assemblies are required to perform most advanced laparoscopic interventions. Trocar-cannula assemblies can be disposable or nondisposable. Typically for veterinary patients, resterilizable nondisposable cannulas are more cost-effective than single-use devices. When 5-mm instrumentation is being used, 6-mm trocar-cannula assemblies are required. Some laparoscopic instruments are 10 mm in diameter (such as some clip appliers, stapling devices, and specimen retrieval bags), so at least one port is established using an 11-mm or 11.5-mm cannula to accommodate a 10-mm instrument. During many advanced procedures, surgical time can be prolonged and many instrument exchanges are performed, so it is helpful to use threaded cannulas rather than smooth ones. Threaded cannulas have the advantage of limiting slippage of the cannula through the body wall, which can be frustrating and can lead to widening of the port incision, leakage of CO_2, and subsequent loss of pneumoperitoneum.

A basic set of laparoscopic instruments are required for all advanced laparoscopic procedures including laparoscopic Metzenbaum scissors, suture-cutting scissors (hook scissors), Kelly forceps, Babcock forceps, cup or punch biopsy forceps, and a blunt probe. In addition, several specialized instruments are required to perform the procedures described in this article. Laparoscopic right-angled forceps are essential for dissection around the cystic duct during cholecystectomy and are helpful for careful dissection of tissue plains in laparoscopic adrenalectomy. Five- and 10-mm right-angled forceps are helpful for cystic duct dissection during cholecystectomy. A laparoscopic retractor is important for numerous applications. Various types and sizes are available, and fan retractors and self-retaining retractors have been reported for use in cholecystectomy and adrenalectomy in dogs.[3,4]

A major challenge in laparoscopic surgery is the ability to achieve excellent hemostasis. Because of the detrimental effect even minor hemorrhage has on visualization of the surgical field, it could be argued that control of minor "nuisance" bleeding is even more important in laparoscopic interventions than in "open" surgery. Various modalities for achieving hemostasis are available. Hemostatic agents such as gelatin sponges (Gelfoam, Pfizer Inc., New York, New York) or oxidized regenerated cellulose (Surgicel, Johnson & Johnson Inc., Paramus, New Jersey) can be passed through a port and manipulated into position for low-grade hemorrhage. Extracorporeal sutures can be used to ligate vessels and other luminal structures such as the common bile duct. When placing extracorporeal sutures, a knot pusher is necessary to push slipknots into position. Laparoscopic clip appliers are also helpful for ligation of vessels and other structures. Many different types are available, but 10-mm clip appliers will usually dispense medium or large clips, and a multifire clip applier reduces the number of instrument exchanges required.

Many cautery modalities are available for use in laparoscopic surgery. Monopolar cautery can be used but is less safe than bipolar energy, as insulation failure, sparking, and direct coupling can all cause damage to adjacent tissues not within the visual field without the surgeon noticing. Several bipolar (Ligasure V, Valleylab Inc., Boulder, Colorado and Enseal Trio, Ethicon Endosurgery Inc., Cinicinnati, Ohio) and ultrasonic (Harmonic Scalpel, Ethicon Endosurgery Inc., Cinicinnati, Ohio) vessel-sealing devices can be used to seal and cut vessels, and having one of these devices available is suggested for surgeons who plan on performing advanced laparoscopic interventions. These devices have been shown to significantly decrease surgical time,[11] and in more advanced procedures reduction in surgical time is likely to be even greater. The devices mentioned all have a fine-tipped version of the handpiece, which is helpful for careful dissection of tissue plains necessary during the procedures described.

Suction-irrigation devices are helpful for aspiration of hemorrhage and fluid accumulations, which improves visualization during the procedure. Nondisposable laparoscopic suction tips are available but can be challenging to regulate precisely. When suction is applied during laparoscopy, CO_2 will also be removed, so short bursts of suction are preferable. Most disposable suction-irrigation devices have buttons allowing fine regulation of the duration and intensity of suction applied. If suction cannot be finely regulated, pneumoperitoneum is rapidly lost with a consequent loss of working space.

Specimen retrieval bags are also necessary when neoplastic or infected tissues are withdrawn through port incisions. Port site metastasis is a well-researched complication of human laparoscopic interventions and has been reported in dogs.[12–14] Specimen retrieval bags are available in many different styles and sizes. Commercially available bags usually come on a 10-mm applicator and are easy to manipulate, but for smaller samples, bags can be made from the body or finger of a sterile surgical glove to reduce cost.

GENERAL TIPS FOR ADVANCED LAPAROSCOPIC TECHNIQUES

Helpful guidelines, if adhered to, can make laparoscopic interventions technically easier for the surgeon, in turn leading to reduced surgical time. These guidelines become especially important when more complex and time-consuming procedures are attempted.

A straight line should always be formed between the location of the surgeon to the lesion or organ operated, and the video monitor. The endoscopy tower is moved accordingly to maintain this straight line. Spatial awareness and hand-eye coordination will be greatly improved by adhering to this principle. Operating room organization has been highlighted for the procedures described later.

There is limited ability in laparoscopic surgery to actively manipulate the position of organs. Gravity can be used to the surgeon's advantage for visualization. The use of either a motorized or manual tilting table can provide a head-down (Trendelenburg), head-up (reverse Trendelenburg), or laterally tilted position, greatly improving visualization of the surgical field by allowing organs to fall away from structures of interest.

An assistant is required for most laparoscopic procedures and will play a major role in the procedure, primarily as the laparoscope operator. The surgeon should always operate both instruments, because two different surgeons using different instruments causes insufficient coordination of movement (just as it would in "open" surgery). The assistant should "drive" the laparoscope and always attempt to minimize motion and maintain a constant view of the surgical field. The surgeon's spatial awareness should enable him or her to "find" the surgical field without the assistant constantly moving the laparoscope to visualize instruments entering through the cannula during instrument exchanges.

LAPAROSCOPIC-ASSISTED CHOLECYSTOSTOMY TUBE PLACEMENT
Indications

Cholecystostomy tubes provide temporary diversion of bile from the gall bladder and aid in the management of extrahepatic biliary tract obstruction (EHBO). The most common causes of EHBO in cats and dogs are pancreatitis and neoplasia; less common causes include cholelithiasis, stricture, and foreign body obstruction.[15–18] Rerouting procedures have traditionally been used to bypass the obstruction but are time consuming, can be associated with various short- and long-term complications, and result in permanent alteration of normal anatomy.[16–19] Options that preserve the normal anatomy of the biliary tree include biliary stenting[20,21] and cholecystostomy tube placement.[22] When potentially reversible disease processes such as pancreatitis occur or patients are judged to be poor candidates for prolonged anesthesia, establishing temporary biliary drainage may be of value. The use of preoperative biliary drainage in high-risk patients before definitive surgical intervention is established in humans, but remains controversial.[23] In small animals with EHBO that are systemically unstable, preoperative drainage allows temporary drainage before definitive surgical intervention. In cases of pancreatitis, cholecystostomy may be therapeutic if the pancreatitis resolves, and bile flow is reestablished and can be documented by cholangiography.

Various techniques are available for placement of cholecystostomy tubes in small animals including the "open" surgical, ultrasound-guided, and laparoscopic-assisted techniques.[22] Laparoscopic-assisted cholecystostomy tube placement has been shown to be technically feasible, and placement is more reliable than with ultrasound guidance, although sucess maybe operator-dependent.[22]

Patient Preparation and Port Placement

Place the dog in dorsal recumbency, and clip and aseptically prepare the abdomen. The surgeon stands on the right side of the dog and the endoscopy tower is placed at the head of the dog on the left side. Establish a subumbilical portal for exploration of the peritoneal cavity. Place one instrument port under direct visualization caudally in the left or right cranial quadrant of the abdomen (the exact location is not critical).

Technique Description

When considering the location for catheter placement, consider where the gall bladder will naturally lie with the dog in a weight-bearing position. This placement will allow the gall bladder to be pulled up and maintained with minimal tension. Catheter entry in a right paraxiphoid position has been reported to have a high success rate.[22] The author has also placed the cholecystostomy tube in a slightly more caudal and right-sided location, just caudal to the costal arch (**Fig. 1**). An 8 to 10 Fr locking loop catheter is normally recommended. Make a stab incision through the skin and use the sharp stylet to penetrate the body wall. Use a blunt probe to manipulate the gall bladder into position to allow the trajectory of the catheter to enter the apex of the gall bladder or to allow passage of the catheter through a section of hepatic parenchyma (**Fig. 2**). The importance of a transhepatic tunnel is debatable. One study found that leak point pressures of nontranshepatically placed cholecystostomy tubes were significantly higher than previously reported intracholic pressures in dogs.[22] The importance of transhepatic passage of the tube in humans also seems to be uncertain.[24] Once the stylet has penetrated the gallbladder it can be withdrawn, ensuring that the catheter is positioned far enough into the gall bladder that all fenestrations are located within the gall bladder. Tighten the string to fix the locking loop in place and prevent catheter migration. Completely empty the gall bladder and gently pull it against the body wall (**Fig. 3**). Use a Chinese finger trap suture to hold the catheter securely in place. Then connect the end of the catheter to a passive, closed collection system.

Complications and Follow-up

The main complications of cholecystostomy tubes are premature obstruction and dislodgment. Obstruction as early as 12 hours postoperatively has been described in a cat.[22] It is likely that thickened, sludgy bile in some gall bladders will not pass

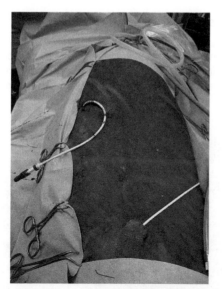

Fig. 1. Postoperative view of a dog with a laparoscopic-assisted cholecystostomy tube in place demonstrating the position of the tube just caudal to the costal arch in the right cranial quadrant. The two small incisions from the camera and instrument portal can also be seen.

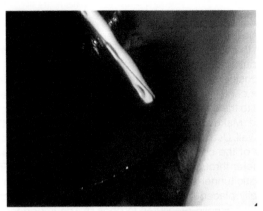

Fig. 2. During laparoscopic-assisted cholecystostomy tube placement, the locking loop catheter can be seen passing transhepatically into the gall bladder.

through the narrow-gauge catheters used without causing obstruction, and it may be helpful to aspirate and flush the catheters on a daily basis; however, care must be taken to prevent ascending infection. Early dislodgment with subsequent intraperitoneal bile leakage has also been reported.[22] Despite some suggestions that 5 to 10 days is sufficient for catheter tract maturation and leakage prevention, recent evidence suggests that maintenance of the catheters for 3 to 4 weeks may be more appropriate.[22] Follow-up cholangiography in cases of pancreatitis or other potentially reversible conditions are performed every 2 to 3 days to evaluate biliary tract patency. If patency is reestablished, the cholecystostomy tube can be capped, wrapped, and left in place for approximately 1 month to prevent leakage. If obstruction remains after 10 to 14 days, consideration should be given to biliary rerouting for long-term biliary drainage.

LAPAROSCOPIC CHOLECYSTECTOMY
Indications

Cholangitis and gallstones are common in people and laparoscopic cholecystectomy (LC) has become a routine procedure in human medicine over the last 30 years. In cats and dogs, conditions treated by cholecystectomy include necrotizing cholecystitis,[25]

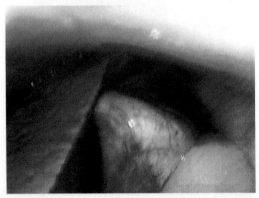

Fig. 3. Once the locking loop has been deployed within the gall bladder, the bile is drained before being pulled up toward the body wall where it is secured on the outside with a Chinese finger trap suture (**Fig. 1**).

gall bladder trauma or neoplasia, symptomatic cholelithiasis,[26,27] and gall bladder mucocele.[28–31] Of these, uncomplicated gall bladder mucoceles are probably the most suitable cases for LC. Although a recent report highlighted the successful medical treatment of two dogs with gall bladder mucocele (GBM),[32] most investigators agree that cholecystectomy is the treatment of choice for GBM, due to the significant morbidity and mortality associated with cases that develop bile peritonitis or EHBO as a consequence. In addition, clinical signs such as vomiting, inappetance, and lethargy can be associated with nonperforated nonobstructive GBMs.[3,31,32]

Another possible indication for LC is symptomatic cholelithiasis without common bile duct stones or associated EHBO, which occurs less frequently. However, care must be taken not to overlook stones that are residing in, or moving into and out of the ductal system.

Contraindications to LC are uncontrolled coagulopathy, the presence of bile peritonitis, extrahepatic biliary tract obstruction, small body size (<4 kg), and the presence of conditions that make a patient poorly tolerant of anesthesia and pneumoperitoneum (such as severe cardiorespiratory diseases and diaphragmatic hernia).

Patient Preparation and Port Placement

Clip the patient from 2.5 to 5 cm (1 to 2 inches) cranial to the xiphoid process to the pubis and laterally to the dorsal third of the abdominal wall. Perform aseptic surgical preparation as for an open surgical approach. Perioperative antibiosis should be used and selected based either on culture and susceptibility testing or on an empiric choice based on the knowledge of commonly encountered hepatobiliary flora. Suitable empiric choices are cefazolin (22 mg/kg IV every 2 h), cefoxitin (22 mg/kg IV every 2 h) or metronidazole (10 mg/kg IV every 2 h). The surgeon should stand on the right side of the patient with the video monitor positioned at the head of the patient on the left side.

A four-port technique is generally used for LC in dogs (**Fig. 4**). Abdominal access should be established using either a Veress needle or the Hasson technique. Establish pneumoperitoneum using a mechanical insufflator making sure that intra-abdominal pressures do not exceed 10 to 12 mmHg. Create a subumbilical port using a trocar-cannula assembly that will allow passage of 10-mm instrumentation. A 5-mm or 10-mm, 0° or 30° laparoscope is inserted into the abdomen, and a full exploration is performed. Insert three 6-mm instrument ports. Port position is as follows: one port 5 to 8 cm lateral and 3 to 5 cm cranial to the umbilicus in the left cranial quadrant, and two ports 3 to 5 and 5 to 8 cm lateral to the umbilicus on the right side in a triangulated pattern around the anticipated location of the gall bladder (**Fig. 4**). These general guidelines may be adapted to accommodate different-sized animals.

Technique Description

Establish good visualization of the area to dissect around the cystic duct. Place the surgical table into a head-down (Trendelenburg) position to allow the liver lobes to move cranially as much as possible. Active retraction of the gall bladder and adjacent liver lobes will be necessary and can be done with a 5-mm fan or other self-retaining retractor through the left-sided instrument port. An assistant manipulates the retractor, and care should be taken not to damage the often friable gall bladder and surrounding hepatic parenchyma. Position the laparoscope in the right-sided instrument port closest to the midline. Right-angled laparoscopic forceps and another dissection instrument such as another right-angled forceps, Kelly forceps, or the vessel-sealing device are placed in the two remaining ports and are operated by the primary surgeon.

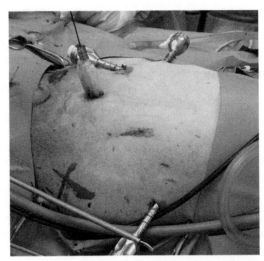

Fig. 4. Port position for laparoscopy is demonstrated with the dog's head located to the right side of the image. The gall bladder now located within the specimen retrieval bag is being pulled out of the subumbilical port incision. The bag will be opened and bile drained before removal from the peritoneal cavity through the port incision.

Once adequate visualization is obtained, use the right-angled forceps to dissect circumferentially around the cystic duct, ensuring that the dissection remains proximal to the entrance of the first hepatic duct to avoid iatrogenic damage. Some hemorrhage is likely, as this dissection proceeds but is typically minor. Use intermittent suction to aspirate hemorrhage and to maintain optimal visualization during the dissection. The dissection is complete when the tips of the right-angled forceps are visible around the cystic duct. Any leakage of bile detected during dissection indicates iatrogenic penetration of the cystic duct, and conversion to an open approach should be considered. The cystic duct can be ligated in a variety of ways. In the case of GBMs, where there is often some thickening and mild distension of the duct, extracorporeal suture placement is recommended.[3] Extracorporeally tied ligatures are tedious to perform but provide good knot security and ensure that the full circumference of the duct has been ligated. Modified Roeder knots of 0 or 2-0 polydioxanone are prepared extracorporeally and pushed into position using a knot pusher.[33] Ideally, three ligatures are placed, and sharp sectioning of the cystic duct is performed with laparoscopic scissors between the two most proximal sutures, leaving one to two ligatures around the cystic duct and one on the gall bladder. It is helpful to leave the end long on the gall bladder suture to aid in manipulation after the cystic duct is transected. Hemostatic clip use is possible in some dogs in which the cystic duct is small and not distended. Medium or large hemostatic clips should be used, and application with a multifire clip applier reduces the number of instrument exchanges. If clips only are used, at least four clips should be applied to the duct before sectioning so that at least two clips remain on each side.

Once the cystic duct is transected, begin dissecting the gall bladder from the hepatic fossa. Upward traction on the gall bladder by manipulation of the suture end or use of a blunt probe is helpful. A vessel-sealing device or bipolar cautery aids in dissection of the gall bladder from the fossa. Once dissected free, place the gall bladder in a specimen retrieval bag inserted through the subumbilical port. Withdraw the entire cannula from the port site with the first part of the retrieval bag (**Fig. 4**).

Place tension on the retrieval bag until a small area of the gall bladder can be visualized and punctured with a number 11 blade, being careful not to penetrate the retrieval bag during the process. Place the tip of the suction device in the gall bladder (which is still located within the abdomen) and suction bile from within the bag. Once the bile has been suctioned completely, pull the empty gall bladder through the telescope port within the specimen retrieval bag. Close the subumbilical port, lavage the gall bladder fossa, and aspirate fluid using the suction-irrigation device. Carefully inspect the hepatic fossa to ensure adequate hemostasis. The gall bladder and a liver biopsy should be submitted for histopathological examination, and bacterial culture and susceptibility testing. Bile should also undergo bacterial culture and sensitivity testing. CO_2 should be purged from the peritoneal cavity before cannula removal and closure of the port sites.

Complications and Follow-up

If significant bile leakage, excessive hemorrhage, or other technical or anesthetic complications occur, conversion to an open approach should be performed. It is not uncommon to see transient elevations in liver enzymes postoperatively.[3] Underlying concurrent hepatobiliary pathology is common, which is why collection of a liver specimen is recommended for hepatobiliary histopathology at the time of LC.[3] Inadequate ligation of the cystic duct causing postoperative bile peritonitis can occur postoperatively. Postoperative EHBO can develop as a result of inadequate flushing of residual biliary sludge in the common bile duct in dogs with GBM. Avoidance of these latter complications is based on careful case selection and the decision not to perform LC in dogs with GBM with preoperative biochemical or imaging evidence of EHBO.

Long-term monitoring and management of associated hepatobiliary disease in patients undergoing LC for GBM or cholelithiasis may be necessary.

LAPAROSCOPIC ADRENALECTOMY
Indications

Laparoscopic adrenalectomy (LA) has been described in people[34,35] and veterinary patients.[4,36] The laparoscopic approach to the adrenal gland in small animals provides excellent visualization for dissection. Appropriate case selection, however, is especially important with LA due to the close anatomic relationship of the glands to large vascular structures and the propensity for these tumors to invade these and other structures. The right adrenal gland is especially challenging, as the gland capsule can be continuous with the tunica externa of the caudal vena cava in dogs, making this dissection challenging, although successful right adrenalectomy has been reported in dogs.[4]

The most common indication for adrenalectomy in small animals is the removal of primary adrenal neoplasms, the most common of which are adrenocortical adenomas, adenocarcinomas, and pheochromocytomas.[37,38] In cats, functional adrenocortical tumors and aldosterone-secreting tumors occur, but are less common.[39–41] Incidentally discovered adrenal masses that do not seem to be associated with specific clinical signs may be detected during routine imaging studies performed for other reasons. Laparoscopic adrenalectomy may provide a less invasive modality for treatment of patients with clinical or incidental masses of the adrenal glands. Every patient, however, should be individually evaluated to decide whether adrenalectomy is warranted based on the clinical signs, presence of comorbidities, and ability to undergo anesthesia, as morbidity and mortality are significant with open and laparoscopic approaches.[4,37,38]

Diagnostic imaging is an important part of the preoperative workup for adrenal masses and forms the basis for decision making as to whether a laparoscopic approach might be feasible. The dimensions of the mass are vital, as are the relationships to surrounding organs and vascular structures. Approximately 25% of adrenal neoplasms exhibit vascular invasion into the vena cava, phrenicoabdominal veins, or renal vasculature, with pheochromocytomas more likely to invade than adrenocortical tumors.[38] If detected preoperatively, vascular invasion should be considered an indication for an "open" approach. Ultrasonography and computed tomography are most often used for preoperative imaging. Ultrasonography has been shown to have a sensitivity and specificity of 80% and 90%, respectively, for detection of tumor thrombus.[38] Sensitivity and specificity of computed tomography or magnetic resonance imaging for detection of vascular invasion are currently unknown, but personal experience with computed tomography has been favorable for detection of the presence and extent of tumor thrombus.

It is suggested that in the early part of the learning curve, animals with functional tumors causing clinical signs or those more than 3 to 4 cm that do not exhibit vascular invasion be considered for LA. Animals that are systemically unstable, have uncontrolled metabolic or acid-base disturbance, uncontrolled coagulopathies, untreated severe arrhythmias, or hypertension should not undergo LA. Animals that may be poorly tolerant of pneumoperitoneum such as those with severe cardiorespiratory disease or those with diaphragmatic herniation are poor candidates.

Vascular invasion of the mass into surrounding vessels or large masses (>6 cm) are indications for open adrenalectomy; however, the effect of tumor size on morbidity during LA has not been evaluated in small animals. Inadequate training or lack of the correct instrumentation is also an important contraindication for LA.

Patient Preparation and Port Placement

Before surgery, the same preoperative management of adrenal neoplasia as would be performed for "open" adrenalectomy should be pursued. In the case of functional adrenocortical tumors, supplementing with corticosteroids before initiation of surgery to avoid a hypoadrenocortical episode in the recovery period is important. Suitable choices include dexamethasone (0.1–0.2 mg/kg IV), prednisolone sodium succinate (1–2 mg/kg IV), or hydrocortisone (2 mg/kg IV). In animals in which pheochromocytoma is suspected, pretreatment with an α-adrenergic blocker, such as phenoxybenzamine, should be considered for several weeks preoperatively until the animal is normotensive, as this drug has been shown to improve outcomes in dogs undergoing adrenalectomy.[42] In cats with functional adrenocortical tumors, it has been suggested that treatment with trilostane be initiated until the skin abnormalities accompanying the condition in this species resolve.[41] Cats with aldosterone-secreting tumors should have their metabolic and electrolyte disturbances corrected before surgery.

In preparation for surgery, liberally clip the hair from 5 cm (2 inches) cranial to the xiphoid process to 2.5 cm (1 inch) caudal to the pubis and laterally to the most dorsal third of the body wall. Carry out a routine aseptic surgical scrub of this entire area, being sure to prepare far enough dorsally as port placement may be dorsal on the affected side. The surgeon should stand on the opposite side of the patient from the adrenal gland being resected, and the video monitor should be placed directly opposite the surgeon.

Appropriate anesthetic management of patients for adrenalectomy is complex and absolutely critical for success. Similar considerations exist for LA as for open adrenalectomy. Readers are directed to standard anesthetic texts for a full discussion of anesthetic management for adrenalectomy.

A three- or four port technique can be used for LA in dogs depending on how much active retraction is necessary. Establish a telescope portal in a subumbilical location using the Hasson technique or a Veress needle. Instrument ports are placed in a triangulating pattern around the location of the adrenal gland (**Fig. 5**). Instruments should not be placed too close together to avoid interference during the dissection. For a left-sided lesion, place a trocar-cannula assembly suitable for passage of 5-mm instrumentation 5 to 10 cm cranial to and 5 to 8 cm lateral to the subumbilical port on the left side in a location just caudal to the costal arch. It is important that the port remain caudal to the last rib to avoid inadvertent penetration of the thoracic cavity. Place a second instrument port 5 to 10 cm caudal and 5 to 8 cm lateral to the subumbilical port in the lower left quadrant. One of these three ports is usually established using a cannula suitable for passage of 10-mm instrumentation, which allows passage of a 10-mm clip applier and specimen retrieval bag. If a right-sided adrenalectomy is being performed, the ports are placed at the same locations but on the opposite side.

Technique Description

Once abdominal access has been achieved, explore the peritoneal cavity to evaluate for intercurrent pathology or signs of metastasis. Closely inspect the liver and biopsy if suspicious lesions are found. Rotate the patient away from the side of the lesion into nearly lateral recumbency. Placement of a small foam wedge under the spine with the animal in lateral recumbency has also been advocated.[4] Obtaining good visualization is the first challenge after port placement for LA. During left-sided LA, the spleen or stomach often obscures visualization of the cranial pole of the adrenal gland, and the kidney sometimes obscures visualization of the caudal margin of the gland. On the right side, the right lateral lobe of the liver must be retracted cranially and the kidney can require retraction dorsally and caudally. Intestines can also intermittently obscure visualization of right or left glands, but will usually fall ventrally once the animal is in lateral recumbency. Several strategies exist for improving visualization. The use of a head-down (Trendelenburg) positioning may prevent the stomach and spleen moving caudally, thus aiding in visualization of the cranial aspects, although this can make visualization of the caudal parts of the dissection more difficult. Alternatively, a third (or more) instrument port(s) can be placed more dorsally over the kidney and a retractor used to move structures cranially or caudally during dissection.[4]

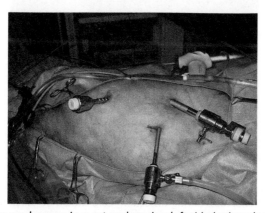

Fig. 5. Port position can be seen in a cat undergoing left-sided adrenalectomy.

In dogs at least part of the adrenal gland is usually visible, allowing the surgeon to initiate dissection of the retroperitoneal space close to the gland. In obese animals and in cats the gland can be completely obscured by fat, in which case dissection through the fat to localize the gland is necessary. Use a vessel-sealing device to cut and coagulate through the tissue planes around the gland. Use a blunt probe or Babcock forceps to aid in manipulation of the gland as the dissection progresses. Intermittent suctioning of small amounts of hemorrhage as well as fat around the gland helps with visualization, and the suction-irrigation tip can be used as an aid to dissection. The adrenal gland receives arterial supply from numerous small arteries and is drained principally by the adrenal vein, which on the right side enters directly into the caudal vena cava and on the left enters the renal vein. Clinically, these smaller vessels are difficult to directly visualize but result in hemorrhage from almost all planes of dissection if a vessel-sealing device or bipolar cautery is not used. The phrenicoabdominal vein and artery are large and must be identified and ligated. Vessel-sealing devices should reliably seal the phrenicoabdominal vessels of small to medium-sized dogs if they are less than 5 to 7 mm in diameter. In larger dogs, place hemoclips on these vessels.

As dissection of the gland progresses, Babcock forceps can sometimes be placed on the tissues surrounding the gland to aid in retraction; however, care should be taken to avoid penetration of the capsule (**Fig. 6**). The gland should be handled with blunt instruments to minimize the risk of penetrating the capsule and tumor seeding of the peritoneal cavity.

To avoid port site metastases, it is important to place the mass in a specimen retrieval bag before removal through the 10-mm port or an enlargement of this port. The surgical site should be thoroughly lavaged with sterile saline and closely inspected for ongoing hemorrhage.

Complications and Follow-up

Several important intraoperative complications are possible during laparoscopic adrenalectomy and are mostly the same as those seen with open adrenalectomy. The ability to address complications may be compromised due to the lack of manual access to the surgical field. Dissection close to major vascular structures makes

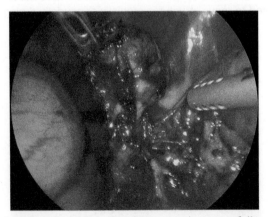

Fig. 6. Laparoscopic Babcock forceps are being used to carefully grasp the tissues surrounding this adrenal mass during dissection. Care should be taken to try not to penetrate the capsule.

profuse hemorrhage possible. If vascular invasion is undetected preoperatively, hemorrhage is more likely to occur, highlighting the importance of preoperative diagnostic imaging. If significant hemorrhage occurs, immediate conversion to an open approach should be performed. If it is possible to suction blood fast enough to visualize a large bleeding vessel clamping or clip application can be performed. The most common problem is "nuisance" hemorrhage that is not hemodynamically significant, but prevents visualization of the surgical field and prolongs surgical time.

Thromboembolism is a potentially fatal complication that has been seen after open[38] and laparoscopic[4] adrenalectomy in dogs, and necessitates careful monitoring for signs of respiratory distress. Preoperative treatment with heparin may reduce the incidence of this problem. In dogs with functional adrenocortical tumors, monitor for postoperative hypoadrenocorticism. Ongoing therapy with corticosteroids should be continued for 2 to 3 weeks postoperatively until the results of adrenocorticotropic hormone (ACTH) stimulation tests confirm normal corticosteroid production from the contralateral adrenal gland. Supplementation with mineralocorticoid (fludrocortisone acetate) is necessary if bilateral adrenalectomy is performed but is not usually necessary after unilateral adrenalectomy.

Most animals with functional adrenocortical tumors will have amelioration of clinical signs postoperatively.[4,37,38] Metastases or intercurrent disease should be considered if clinical signs do not abate. Confirmation of normal adrenal function in previously hyperadrenocortical animals should be performed several weeks after surgery using the ACTH stimulation test.

SUMMARY

As more surgeons perform greater numbers of laparoscopic interventions, the complexity of these interventions will naturally increase. The procedures described are technically demanding and should be performed by surgeons with experience of laparoscopic procedures and with experience of performing those procedures in an "open" fashion. Once mastered, these procedures will add to the ever-growing armamentarium of minimally invasive interventions that have the potential to significantly decrease associated morbidities in small animal patients.

REFERENCES

1. Livingston EH, Rege RV. A nationwide study of conversion from laparoscopic to open cholecystectomy. Am J Surg 2004;188:205–11.
2. Brasesco OE, Rosin D, Rosenthal RJ. Laparoscopic surgery of the liver and biliary tract. J Laparoendosc Adv Surg Tech A 2002;12:91–100.
3. Mayhew PD, Mehler SJ, Radhakrishnan A. Laparoscopic cholecystectomy of uncomplicated gall bladder mucocele in six dogs. Vet Surg 2008;37:625–30.
4. Pelaez MJ, Bouvy BM, Dupre GP. Laparoscopic adrenalectomy for treatment of unilateral adrenocortical carcinomas: techniques, complications and results in seven dogs. Vet Surg 2008;37:444–53.
5. Schirmer BD, Edge SB, Dix JD, et al. Laparoscopic cholecystectomy. Ann Surg 1991;213:665–76.
6. Lee J, El-Tamer M, Schifftner T, et al. Open and laparoscopic adrenalectomy: analysis of the national surgical quality improvement program. J Am Coll Surg 2008;206:953–9.
7. Walsh PJ, Remedios AM, Ferguson JF, et al. Thoracoscopic versus open partial pericardectomy in dogs: comparison of post-operative pain and morbidity. Vet Surg 1999;28:472–9.

8. Devitt CM, Cox RE, Hailey JJ. Duration, complications, stress and pain of open ovariohysterectomy versus a simple method of laparoscopic-assisted ovariohysterectomy in dogs. J Am Vet Med Assoc 2005;227:921–7.

9. Culp WTN, Mayhew PD, Brown DC. The effect of laparoscopic versus open ovariectomy on post-operative activity in small dogs. In: Proceedings of the 2008 ACVS Veterinary Symposium. San Diego; 2008. p. 6.

10. Mayhew PD, Brown DC. Prospective evaluation of two intracorporeally-sutured laparoscopic gastropexy techniques compared to laparoscopic-assisted gastropexy in dogs. In: Proceedings of the 2008 ACVS Veterinary Symposium. San Diego; 2008. p. 22.

11. Mayhew PD, Brown DC. Comparison of three techniques for ovarian pedicle hemostasis during laparoscopic-assisted ovariohysterectomy. Vet Surg 2007; 36:541–7.

12. Ramirez PT, Wolf JK, Levenback C. Laparoscopic port-site metastases: etiology and prevention. Gynecol Oncol 2003;91:179–89.

13. Curet MJ. Port site metastases. Am J Surg 2004;187:705–12.

14. Brisson BA, Reggeti F, Bienzle D. Portal site metastasis of invasive mesothelioma after diagnostic thoracoscopy in a dog. J Am Vet Med Assoc 2006;229:980–3.

15. Fahie M, Martin RA. Extrahepatic biliary tract obstruction: a retrospective study of 45 cases (1983–1993). J Am Anim Hosp Assoc 1995;31:478–82.

16. Mayhew PD, Holt DE, McLear RC, et al. Pathogenesis and outcome of extrahepatic biliary obstruction in cats. J Small Anim Pract 2002;43:247–53.

17. Mehler SJ, Mayhew PD, Drobatz KJ, et al. Variables associated with outcome in dogs undergoing extrahepatic biliary surgery: 60 cases (1988–2002). Vet Surg 2004;33:644–9.

18. Buote NJ, Mitchell SL, Penninck D, et al. Cholecystoenterostomy for treatment of extrahepatic biliary tract obstruction in cats: 22 cases (1994–2003). J Am Vet Med Assoc 2006;228:1376–82.

19. Matthiesen DT. Complications associated with surgery of the extrahepatic biliary system. Probl Vet Med 1989;1:295–313.

20. Mayhew PD, Richardson RW, Mehler SJ, et al. Choledochal tube stenting for decompression of the extrahepatic portion of the biliary tract in dogs:13 cases (2002–2005). J Am Vet Med Assoc 2006;228:1209–14.

21. Mayhew PD, Weisse CW. Treatment of pancreatitis-associated extrahepatic biliary tract obstruction by choledochal stenting in seven cats. J Small Anim Pract 2008;49:133–8.

22. Murphy SM, Rodriguez JD, McAnulty JF. Minimally invasive cholecystostomy in the dog: evaluation of placement techniques and use in extrahepatic biliary obstruction. Vet Surg 2007;36:675–83.

23. Sewnath ME, Karsten TM, Prins MH, et al. A meta-analysis on the efficacy of preoperative biliary drainage for tumors causing obstructive jaundice. Ann Surg 2002;236:17–27.

24. Garber SJ, Mathleson JR, Cooperberg PL, et al. Percutaneous cholecystostomy: safety of the transperitoneal route. J Vasc Interv Radiol 1994;5:295–8.

25. Church EM, Matthiesen DT. Surgical treatment of 23 dogs with necrotizing cholecystitis. J Am Anim Hosp Assoc 1988;24:305–10.

26. Kirpensteijn J, Fingland RB, Ulrich T, et al. Cholelithiasis in dogs: 29 cases (1980–1990). J Am Vet Med Assoc 1993;202:1137–42.

27. Eich CS, Ludwig LL. The surgical treatment of cholelithiasis in cats: a study of nine cases. J Am Anim Hosp Assoc 2002;38:290–6.

28. Besso JG, Wrigley RH, Gliatto JM, et al. Ultrasonographic appearance and clinical findings in 14 dogs with gallbladder mucocele. Vet Radiol Ultrasound 2000; 41:261–71.
29. Pike FS, Berg J, King NW, et al. Gall bladder mucocele in dogs: 30 cases (2000–2002). J Am Vet Med Assoc 2004;224:1615–22.
30. Worley DR, Hottinger HA, Lawrence HJ. Surgical management of gallbladder mucoceles in dogs: 22 cases (1999–2003). J Am Vet Med Assoc 2004;225:1418–22.
31. Aguirre AL, Center SA, Randolph JF, et al. Gallbladder disease in Shetland Sheepdogs: 38 cases (1995–2005). J Am Vet Med Assoc 2007;231:79–88.
32. Walter R, Dunn ME, d'Anjou MA, et al. Nonsurgical resolution of gallbladder mucocele in two dogs. J Am Vet Med Assoc 2008;232:1688–93.
33. Stoloff DR. Laparoscopic suturing and knot tying techniques. In: Freeman LJ, editor. Veterinary endosurgery. 1st edition. St Louis (MO): Mosby Inc; 1999. p. 73–91.
34. David G, Yoav M, Gross D, et al. Laparoscopic adrenalectomy: ascending the learning curve. Surg Endosc 2004;18:771–3.
35. Gil-Cardenas A, Cordon C, Gamino R, et al. Laparoscopic adrenalectomy: lessons learned from an initial series of 100 patients. Surg Endosc 2008;22: 991–5.
36. Freeman LJ. Minimally invasive adrenalectomy. In: Freeman LJ, editor. Veterinary endosurgery. 1st edition. St Louis (MO): Mosby Inc; 1999. p. 199–203.
37. Anderson CR, Birchard SJ, Powers BE, et al. Surgical treatment of adrenocortical tumors: 21 cases (1990–1996). J Am Anim Hosp Assoc 2001;37:93–7.
38. Kyles AE, Feldman EC, De Cock HEV, et al. Surgical management of adrenal gland tumors with and without associated tumor thrombi in dogs: 40 cases. J Am Vet Med Assoc 2003;223:654–62.
39. Duesberg CA, Nelson RW, Feldman EC, et al. Adrenalectomy for treatment of hyperadrenocorticism in cats: 10 cases (1988–1992). J Am Vet Med Assoc 1995; 207:1066–70.
40. Ash RA, Harvey AM, Tasker S. Primary hyperaldosteronism in the cat: a series of 13 cases. J Feline Med Surg 2005;7:173–82.
41. Chiaramonte D, Greco DS. Feline adrenal disorders. Clin Tech Small Anim Pract 2007;22:26–31.
42. Herrera MA, Mehl ML, Kass PH, et al. Predictive factors and the effect of phenoxybenzamine on outcome in dogs undergoing adrenalectomy for pheochromocytoma. J Vet Intern Med 2008;22:1333–9.

Complications and Need for Conversion to Laparotomy in Small Animals

Janet Kovak McClaran, DVM*, Nicole J. Buote, DVM

KEYWORDS

- Laparoscopy • Complications • Conversion
- Pneumoperitoneum • Contraindications

Laparoscopic procedures performed in veterinary medicine include diagnostic and therapeutic procedures. Diagnostic procedures may include biopsies of almost any abdominal organ including the liver, spleen, lymph nodes, kidney, pancreas, and gastrointestinal tract. Therapeutic procedures that have been documented in small animal medicine include feeding tube placement, gastropexy, ovariohysterectomy, ovariectomy, cryptorchidectomy, cholecystostomy catheter placement, adrenalectomy, and cholecystectomy.[1–11] Laparoscopic procedures provide the advantage of decreased patient morbidity with improved visualization and fast patient recovery. Limitations of laparoscopy include the time and cost associated with training and equipment maintenance. Complications associated with laparoscopic procedures may be categorized as intraoperative and postoperative. Conversion to laparotomy, although not always a complication, may be classified as elective or emergent. Conversion rates in humans vary depending on a variety of patient-, procedure-, and surgeon-related factors. There are few contraindications for performing laparoscopic procedures, but complications or conversions to an open laparotomy may be expected in a percentage of patients.

COMPLICATIONS ASSOCIATED WITH LAPAROSCOPY

Complications associated with laparoscopy may be anticipated in a small number of patients. Overall rates of complications in human medicine vary widely depending on procedures performed. The complication rate of laparoscopic procedures has previously been sited as low as 2% in one veterinary text but has never been specifically studied.[1] Complications may be divided into major and minor complications as well as those encountered during surgery and those that may be anticipated

---

Department of Surgery, The Animal Medical Center, 510 East 62nd Street, New York, NY 10065, USA
* Corresponding author.
E-mail address: janet.mcclaran@amcny.org (J.K. McClaran).

Vet Clin Small Anim 39 (2009) 941–951
doi:10.1016/j.cvsm.2009.05.003
0195-5616/09/$ – see front matter © 2009 Elsevier Inc. All rights reserved.

postoperatively. Complications may be associated with anesthesia and maintenance of a pneumoperitoneum, equipment malfunction, and trocar insertion, as well as organ manipulation and biopsy. Following completion of surgery, complications may arise with hemorrhage, peritonitis, port site incisions, or adhesion formation. **Table 1** outlines potential complications that may be encountered with laparoscopy. As the number of procedures being performed increases, one can anticipate the reported complication levels may also increase.

PNEUMOPERITONEUM

Reported anesthetic complications associated with laparoscopy usually involve patients' inability to tolerate pneumoperitoneum. Hypercarbia or hypoxia are generally encountered in patients with a history of preexisting pulmonary or cardiac disease.[12] The cardiopulmonary effects of carbon dioxide insufflation for the establishment of a pneumoperitoneum have been determined. Abdominal insufflation using CO_2 to a pressure of 15 mmHg for 180 minutes resulted in significant increases in heart rate, minute ventilation, and saphenous vein pressure, and decreases in pH and PaO_2.[13] These changes, however, were found to be acceptable in healthy, well-ventilated dogs.[13] Serious anesthetic complications include death, and air or CO_2 embolism.[14,15] Careful monitoring of carbon dioxide tension and ventilation minute volume is required to identify patients that develop CO_2 embolism, which occurs by direct injection of CO_2 into the venous system through a Veress needle. Patients become profoundly hypotensive, cyanotic, bradycardic, or develop asystole. Treatment includes cessation of insufflation, delivery of 100% oxygenation, placement of the patient in steep left lateral Trendelenburg position, and placement of a central line to aspirate gas from the venous system.[16] Tension pneumothorax has been reported in patients with a congenital or iatrogenic diaphragmatic defect.[17] Other reported complications following CO_2 pneumoperitoneum include signs of reperfusion injury and peritoneal acidosis, which may lead to attenuation of the inflammatory response after laparoscopic surgery.[18,19]

OPERATIVE COMPLICATIONS

Operative complications may be related to equipment malfunction and level of surgeon experience. The most common complications are encountered with trocar

Table 1 Potential complications with laparoscopy	
Intraoperative	**Postoperative**
Excessive hemorrhage	Incisional (subcutaneous emphysema, seroma, dehiscence, hernia, infection)
Penetration of hollow viscus	Peritonitis
Anesthetic complication (hypotension, cardiovascular compromise)	Anemia (requiring transfusions)
Equipment malfunction	Hypotension requiring treatment
Pulmonary complication (air embolus)	Pulmonary complication (air embolus)
Loss of insufflation	Port site metastasis
—	Adhesion formation

and portal placement.[20] The closed technique uses a Veress needle for insufflation followed by blind insertion of a sharp trocar and cannula. Damage may include minimal hemorrhage, but major complications including major vessel rupture, urinary bladder damage, gastrointestinal tract perforation, and splenic laceration may be encountered. A safer approach to trocar placement is the open, or Hasson, technique, which involves making a small subumbilical incision under direct visualization followed by insertion of a blunt cannula trocar and cannula. A study of 40 horses examined the safety of a variety of trocar placement techniques and found that problems with insufflation or cannula insertion occurred in 12 horses.[21] Complications included peritoneal detachment, splenic puncture, and descending colon perforation. These complications were significantly more frequent with the Veress technique than with open techniques that allowed for direct visualization and insertion of a cannula.[21] Minor lacerations may be successfully repaired with intracorporeal suturing, but most cases of perforation require conversion to an open laparotomy. A serious complication may occur if injuries to bowel or vasculature are not recognized at the time of trocar insertion and hemoabdomen, peritonitis, or abscessation occurs.[17] **Box 1** outlines measures that may be taken to decrease risks associated with trocar placement. Newer, self-dilating, and "optical" trocars allow direct visualization through each abdominal layer, and have been associated with fewer reported complications.[16] A prospective study of 14,243 laparoscopic procedures performed on human patients documented an incidence of trocar-related vascular and visceral injury in 0.18% of patients. These injuries were repaired laparoscopically in 21.7% of patients and by way of laparotomy in 78.2% of individuals. Only one death was reported related to trocar injury.[16]

Other major complications that may occur during laparoscopic procedures include damage to viscera during organ manipulation and hemorrhage following organ biopsy. Hemorrhage following diagnostic liver biopsies in human medicine is rare and has been reported to be 1.3% in a study of 603 patients that underwent diagnostic laparoscopy.[22] In a study of 45 small animal patients that underwent liver biopsy at our facility, 6 animals (18.8%) that were not anemic before surgery were considered anemic following liver biopsy; however, the mean drop in packed cell volume (PCV) was only 2% in these patients. Two of the 45 dogs (4.4%) in the study required a blood transfusion. Only 1 dog (2.2%) required conversion to laparotomy for definitive mass excision and no fatalities were associated with laparoscopic liver biopsy.[4]

The optimal jaw size of laparoscopic graspers has been studied to minimize iatrogenic damage to viscera.[23] With increasing jaw size, the contact area with tissue

---

Box 1
Avoiding iatrogenic trocar insertion complications

- Empty bladder before procedure
- Place animal in slight Trendelenburg (head-down) position
- Hasson technique
- Ensure adequate insufflation
- Aim first trocar toward right cranial quadrant
- Plan subsequent portal sites with transillumination
- Place instrument portals under direct visualization
- Fully inspect abdomen before closure

increases and the pinch force leading to tissue damage decreases. Therefore the optimal jaw has a large contact area to prevent tissue damage as well as a profile that prevents tissue from slipping.[23] Thermal bowel injury may also occur following use of electrosurgical or electrocautery devices.[16] Occurrence of this complication has been reported to be 0.2%.[16] The true incidence of this and other complications is difficult to access due to underreporting. For example, a survey at an American College of Surgeons meeting reported that 18% of respondents had had an inadvertent laparoscopic cautery injury occur in their practice, but 54% of these individuals knew of at least one other surgeon who had experienced such an event.[16]

POSTOPERATIVE COMPLICATIONS

Following the completion of laparoscopic procedures, reported complications documented in the human literature include postoperative hemorrhage, anastomotic leakage, subcutaneous emphysema, persistent pneumoperitoneum, and portal site inflammation, infection, or herniation.[17,22] Major complications are generally classified as those requiring additional surgery or transfusion. In a prospective study of 603 human patients undergoing diagnostic laparoscopic procedures, liver biopsy was the most common procedure leading to major hemorrhage and occurred in 1.3% of patients.[22] Perforation of the gastrointestinal tract requiring an additional procedure occurred in 0.6% of patients. Minor complications occurred in 5.1% of patients and included port site leakage of ascites, cellulitis, hematoma, and wound dehiscence. The overall mortality rate following laparoscopic procedures in this study was 0.49%.[22]

Late complications related to portal site include herniation, infection, and port site metastasis.[24–26] Herniation of omentum through 5-mm laparoscopic port sites in dogs has been reported.[27] It is important to ensure all abdominal organs and fat are adequately within the abdomen as ports are removed, and the fascial layer should be closed under direct visualization. To reduce wound complications following laparoscopic procedures, as with open laparotomy, animals should be adequately exercise restricted with Elizabethan collars, and owners instructed to monitor incision sites daily.

Many theories exist for the formation of port site metastasis and include direct implantation during sample retrieval, exfoliation of cells during tumor manipulation, and dispersion following CO_2 insufflation or by hematogenous spread.[28,29] Controversy exists as to whether higher rates occur following laparoscopy or laparotomy. A study surveying 607 human surgeons who reported on a total of 117,840 total patients undergoing laparoscopic procedures reported an overall rate of tumor reoccurrence in 0.09% of cases, regardless of whether specimen retrieval bags were used.[30] A study comparing laparoscopy to laparotomy found there was no evidence of an increase in circulating tumor cells following laparoscopy, but use of specimen retrieval bags for exteriorization of tumor samples is still recommended.[31]

Identifying patients that are more likely to have a complication associated with a laparoscopic procedure may be useful. In the human literature complications are usually specific to procedure type. A study of 1316 human patients who underwent elective laparoscopic colorectal procedures attempted to identify risk factors for intra- and postoperative complications.[25] Older patients and those with malignant neoplasia were more likely to suffer an intraoperative complication, and male gender, increasing age, increasing American Society of Anesthesiologists (ASA) score, malignant neoplasia, and experience level of the surgeon were all associated with the frequency of encountering a postoperative complication.[25]

Only a few veterinary studies report postoperative complications such as subcutaneous cellulitis, respiratory compromise, suture reaction, fever, and bruising, but risk factors for complications have never been discussed due to their mostly minor nature and small case numbers.[8,10] One report did look at preoperative, intraoperative, and postoperative factors associated with complication rate in a large population of patients.[5] Pre- and postoperative factors and surgical findings were also compared with outcome, including length of stay and survival to discharge.[5]

Results of Retrospective Study

There were 56 canines and 40 felines enrolled in the study.[5] Out of this population, 42 laparoscopic liver biopsies (including those patients that also had splenic biopsies), 52 abdominal explorations with multiple organ samples taken (including but not limited to liver, stomach, intestines, and lymph nodes), 1 laparoscopic assisted gastropexy, and 1 laparoscopic ovariectomy were performed during the study period. Thirty-four out of 96 (35%) patients had complications while in the hospital. Major complications were defined as those cases of intraoperative hemorrhage requiring emergent conversion or postoperative transfusion, or those resulting in an intraoperative death. Six patients had major intraoperative hemorrhage requiring conversion: 2 were trocar-related bleeding injuries and 4 were due to biopsy site bleeding. Postoperative blood transfusions were required in 11 patients; 2 of these were cases of intraoperative hemorrhage and conversion, 4 were anemic preoperatively and had no evidence of bleeding or complications intraoperatively, and 5 were not anemic preoperatively with no evidence of bleeding at surgery. The other patients had minor complications including one involving intraoperative equipment malfunction, 3 patients that developed a seroma at a portal site, 6 with mild postoperative anemia, and 17 requiring treatment of hypotension. The individual significant factors for each complication are detailed in **Table 2**. There were no significant associations between the presenting clinical signs and intraoperative or postoperative complications.

There was a significantly increased likelihood of complications in feline patients, older patients, and patients with lower body condition score and weight. As is the case with the individual complications, lower body weight (kg) and body condition score may make the procedure more technically difficult, leading to iatrogenic trauma; these patients may be undernourished due to their primary disease and older patients may not be able to compensate as well as younger animals during anesthesia. There were significantly increased numbers of postoperative complications in those surgeries supervised by a board-certified surgeon (42%) compared with those without (19%). This result is most likely due to a bias toward board-certified surgeons to perform more difficult surgeries than their less experienced counterparts. There was no significant association between the diagnosis of neoplasia and postoperative complications, but length of hospitalization was significantly increased by the presence of complications. Due to the small number (5 of 96) of patients that did not survive to discharge,

Table 2			
Significant factors related to postoperative complications			
Anemia	**Transfusions**	**Hypotension**	**Any Complication**
• Presence of ascites	• Male gender	• Feline	• Feline
• Conversion	• Ascites	• Conversions	• Increasing age
• Previous abdominal surgery	• Low body condition score	• Low body weight	• Low body condition score
			• Supervision by American College of Veterinary Surgeons diplomate

no significant associations could be made between outcome and any postoperative complications.

In conclusion, the authors found that 35% of patients had some type of complication postoperatively; only 6% of all patients were considered to have a major complication. Felines, patients with lower body condition scores, surgeries resulting in conversions, and older subjects and those of lighter weight were significantly more likely to incur postsurgical complications.

CONVERSION TO LAPAROTOMY

Conversion from laparoscopy to laparotomy alone is not a complication. In human medicine, conversion rates and risk factors have been specifically calculated for the most common laparoscopic procedures, such as cholecystectomy (1%–10%), colorectal procedures (1%–40%), nephrectomy (5%–14%), adrenalectomy (0%–20%), and splenectomy (1%–18%).[9,11,24,32,33] An elective conversion is defined as a case that is converted to a laparotomy in the absence of a complication. An emergent conversion is defined as a case that must be converted due to the development of a complication that cannot be adequately managed using laparoscopy.[12] Although conversion is not always a complication, those patients that undergo a laparotomy may have an increased requirement for intensive care.[33] It is important to recognize when the technical limitations of a laparoscopic procedure have been exceeded. Belizon and colleagues[34] showed that conversions performed within the first 30 minutes of an operation have a better clinical outcome than conversions performed later in a procedure, therefore elective conversions should have a set time limit for the laparoscopic procedures.

Elective conversions are those cases that are converted due to factors that preclude safe and timely laparoscopic completion of procedures. Failure to progress occurs due to factors including adhesions from prior procedures, poor exposure (for reasons such as patient obesity, aberrant or unclear anatomy), or surgeon inexperience. Emergent conversions require immediate conversion to an open laparotomy and include cases of uncontrollable bleeding or rupture of a hollow viscus. Conversions may be classified in multiple ways, but in most cases conversions can be classified as those relating to patient-specific, procedure-specific, or surgeon-specific factors.

Patient-specific factors include patient age, gender, body mass index, individual disease, and anatomic variations. Age has been found to be of variable significance in many human studies for patients undergoing laparoscopic colorectal surgical procedures and cholecystectomy; however, an age younger than 55 and 65 years old, respectively, has been protective.[12,35] Obesity, defined as a body mass index of more than 30 or approximately 22.7 kg (50 pounds) more than ideal body weight, is a risk factor with biliary and colorectal surgeries, and leads to difficulty in proper port placement, and problems with visualization and maneuverability due to intra-abdominal adipose tissue.[12,35–37] Reasons for conversion may also include inappropriate case selection. Large, invasive, or adherent tumors may exceed the limits of what can safely be removed using laparoscopy. Procedure-related reasons for conversion are related to the specific type of procedure being performed as well as intraoperative findings such as adhesions or infection. Other procedural variables include technical problems such as instrument malfunction or problems in maintaining insufflation. In addition, anesthesia-related issues may be a cause for conversion, such as poor patient tolerance of a pneumoperitoneum leading to hypercarbia or hypoxemia. Finally, surgeon-specific factors contributing to conversion rates include level of experience and number of prior procedures performed.[5,6,8,9] A lack of surgeon experience

(<50 cases) has been significant for higher conversion rates in human colorectal surgeries, and it is recommended that surgeons choose uncomplicated cases initially.[12,38]

The most common indications for conversion in human medicine are outlined in **Table 3** and are divided into those for elective or emergent conversions.[12] These classifications do not currently exist in veterinary surgery. One report did look at preoperative, intraoperative, and postoperative factors associated with complication rate in a large population of patients.[5] Pre- and postoperative factors and surgical findings were also compared with outcome, including length of stay and survival to discharge.

Results of Retrospective Study

There were 56 canines and 40 felines enrolled in the study.[5] Out of this population, 42 laparoscopic liver biopsies (including those patients that also had splenic biopsies), 52 abdominal explorations with multiple organ samples taken (including but not limited to liver, stomach, intestines, and lymph nodes), 1 laparoscopic assisted gastropexy, and 1 laparoscopic ovariectomy were performed during the study period. Twenty-two of these patients (23%) underwent an emergent or elective conversion. There were 15 of 22 (68%) elective conversions performed and 7 of 22 (32%) emergent conversions. The most common reason for any conversion was inability to retrieve the desired sample, seen in 12 of 22 (54%) patients. Elective conversions were most often performed due to inability to retrieve the sample (11 of 15, 73%) but occasionally due to inadequate visualization from adhesions (4 of 15, 27%). None of the cases were converted due to inadequate exposure of the organ of interest by excessive intra-abdominal adipose/omental tissue. Of the 7 cases of emergent conversions, 6 were due to excessive bleeding; the seventh was converted due to a biliary tract rupture during manipulation. The reasons for conversion are listed in **Table 4**.

There was no significant difference between converted patients and those not converted with regard to preoperative variables. Solitary liver disease was found to be highly associated with conversion, as 8 of 16 cases (50%) of these patients needed conversion, whereas only 13 of 68 (17%) without this finding required conversion ($P<.01$). The sensitivity and specificity of a solitary liver tumor as a predictive factor was 50% and 83%, respectively. It is generally agreed that laparotomy provides easier access for removal of a solitary hepatic tumor, but laparoscopy may be performed before laparotomy to determine if the lesion is resectable or if the disease is metastatic. Analysis of preoperative blood work values and association with conversion

Table 3	
Potential reasons for conversion	
Elective	**Emergent**
Adhesions from prior surgery	Severe bleeding
Adhesions from inflammatory disease	Injury to hollow viscus
Visualization obscured due to excessive intra-abdominal adipose tissue	Anesthetic complications requiring conversion (hypercarbia, hypoxia)
Poor insufflation	—
Aberrant anatomy	—
Inability to retrieve sample	—
Technical malfunction	—

Table 4 Conversion percentages of unpublished data[5]	
Reason	**Percentage**
Inability to retrieve sample	54 (12/22)
Excessive hemorrhage	27 (6/22)
Intra-abdominal adhesions (inadequate visualization)	23 (5/22)
Rupture of hollow viscus (gallbladder)	4.5 (1/22)

revealed that only 11% of patients with a high level of total solids (more than the median value of 7.0 g/dL) versus 33% of those patients with a low total solids level were converted ($P = .03$). The sensitivity and specificity of preoperative low total solids level as a predictive factor was 89% and 67%, respectively. A low total solids level may be associated with decreased nutritional intake, intestinal inflammatory diseases, renal disease, or decreased hepatic function, which may be associated with an increased chance of bleeding or difficulty removing samples if the tissue is inflamed; however, this association is tenuous.

The histologic diagnosis of neoplasia after surgery was significantly associated with conversion ($P<.01$) as is the case in human studies.[33] The sensitivity and specificity of neoplasia as a predictive factor was 64% and 89%, respectively. The size and invasiveness of the tumor are major factors for conversion in human studies as is the histologic type due to fears of port site metastasis, which was not observed in this report. There was no significant association between conversions and supervision by a board-certified surgeon (22% nonboarded; 23% diplomate) or timing of the procedure early in the course of the study (between 2004 and 2006) and late in the study (2007–2008) with 22% and 24% conversion rate, respectively, most likely due to case selection. There were no statistically significant associations between any factors and the type of conversion (elective versus emergent) due to the small numbers in each group, so this line of enquiry should be explored in the future.

There was no significant difference in survival or length of hospitalization between the groups (82% of patients in the converted group survived to discharge; 99% of patients in the nonconverted group).[5] Overall, there was a survival to discharge of 95% for the entire study population. The major limitation of this study was its retrospective nature and an important limitation was the inclusion of multiple types of procedure. Conversion rates for laparoscopy have not been widely reported in the veterinary literature, so although the risk factors for conversions of diverse procedures may be different, there may be some universally important variables.[12,38] In conclusion, a conversion rate of 23% was found in the population of patients undergoing a laparoscopic procedure and a preoperative finding of a solitary liver tumor, low total solids level, and a diagnosis of malignancy were all significant risk factors for conversion.

CONTRAINDICATIONS

Contraindications for laparoscopy are an important consideration in planning these procedures and in human medicine there are clearly defined limitations.[38] Patient-specific contraindications can include anatomic considerations as well as physiologic abnormalities. Anatomic considerations reported as potential contraindications include adhesions from previous abdominal surgery, intraperitoneal mesh or implants, liver disease leading to ascites, peritonitis, mechanical bowel obstructions, disseminated neoplasia due to the possibility port site recurrence, and invasive cancers.[12,38] Physiologic considerations that may make laparoscopy unsafe include pregnancy,

Table 5 Potential contraindications to laparoscopy	
Relative	**Definitive**
Older patients	Peritonitis[a]
Low body condition score	Diffuse neoplasia[a]
Low total solids	Mechanical bowel obstruction[a]
Previous intra-abdominal surgery (including implantation of mesh)[a]	Pregnancy[a]
Coagulopathies[a]	Intracranial disease[a]
Cardiac/respiratory/liver disease[a]	—

[a] Considered a human contraindication as well.

increased intracranial pressure, cardiac output abnormalities, gas exchange irregularities, liver disease, and coagulopathies.[38]

In veterinary medicine, contraindications have been considered relative and include ascites, coagulopathies, and poor patient condition.[1] In a retrospective study of laparoscopic procedures, felines, patients with lower body condition scores, and older subjects were significantly more likely to incur postsurgical complications.[5] These factors may be considered relative contraindications but many types of procedure were included in this study and older patients with poor body condition scores may be predisposed to complications regardless of the procedure type.[5] Contraindications should not be confined to those conditions that may make laparoscopy unsafe for the patient but also include those conditions or factors that would lead to a high rate of conversion. Inadequate training and experience has been one of the most important limitations to laparoscopy in human medicine but was not found to be associated with a higher rate of conversion or complications in a large retrospective animal study.[5] In conclusion, a modified list of potential contraindications to laparoscopy has been created (**Table 5**), which should help practitioners make appropriate surgical decisions. Every case should be considered individually and the best possible plan created, realizing all potential complications and outcomes.

SUMMARY

In the veterinary literature only small case series or case reports have been published relating to laparoscopic techniques. Intraoperative complication rates range from 2% to 35%, with the majority reported to consist of minor bleeding.[5,7–11,39,40] A conversion rate of 23% has been reported, and elective and emergent conversions during laparoscopic procedures can be expected. Identifying patient, disease, or procedural factors that may predict complications and the need for conversion to a laparotomy may help define future criteria and contraindications for patient selection.

REFERENCES

1. Tweet DC, Monnet E. Laparoscopy: technique and clinical experience. In: McCarthy TC, editor. Veterinary endoscopy for the small animal practitioner. Philadelphia: Elsevier; 2005. p. 357–86.
2. Murphy SM, Rodriguez JD, McAnulty JF. Minimally invasive cholecystostomy in the dog: evaluation of placement techniques and use in extrahepatic biliary obstruction. Vet Surg 2007;36(7):675–83.

3. Rawlings CA, Mahaffey MB, Bement S, et al. Prospective evaluation of laparoscopic-assisted gastropexy in dogs susceptible to gastric dilatation. J Am Vet Med Assoc 2002;221(11):1576–81.

4. Koprowski AC, Kovak JR, Monette S, et al. Evaluation of laparoscopic hepatic biopsy specimens in dogs and cats. In: Proceedings of the 4th Annual Meeting of the Veterinary Endoscopy Society. Hawk's Cay; 2007. p. 8.

5. Buote NJ, Kovak JR. Indications and occurrence of conversion from laparoscopy to laparotomy. In: Proceedings of the 5th Annual Meeting of the Veterinary Endoscopic Society. Keystone; 2008. p. 12.

6. Chandler JC, Kudnig ST, Monnet E. Use of laparoscopic-assisted jejunostomy for fecal diversion in the management of a rectocutaneous fistula in a dog. J Am Vet Med Assoc 2005;226(5):746–51.

7. Devitt CM, Cox RE, Hailey JJ. Duration, complications, stress, and pain of open ovariohysterectomy versus a simple method of laparoscopic-assisted ovariohysterectomy in dogs. J Am Vet Med Assoc 2005;227(6):921–7.

8. Pelaez MJ, Bouvy BM, Dupre GP. Laparoscopic adrenalectomy for treatment of unilateral adrenocortical carcinomas: technique, complications, and results in 7 dogs. Vet Surg 2008;37:444–53.

9. Hewitt SA, Brisson BA, Sinclair MD, et al. Evaluation of laparoscopic-assisted placement of jejunostomy feeding tubes in dogs. J Am Vet Med Assoc 2004; 225:65–71.

10. Davidson EB, Moll HD, Payton ME. Comparison of laparoscopic ovariohysterectomy and ovariohysterectomy in dogs. Vet Surg 2004;33:62–9.

11. Mayhew PD, Mehler SJ, Radhakrishnan A. Laparoscopic cholecystectomy for management of uncomplicated gall bladder mucocele in six dogs. Vet Surg 2008;37:625–30.

12. Halpin VJ, Soper NJ. Decision to convert to open methods. In: Whelan RL, Fleshman JW, Fowler DL, editors. The SAGES manual perioperative care in minimally invasive surgery. New York: Springer; 2006. p. 296–306.

13. Duke T, Steinacher SL, Remedios AM. Cardiopulmonary effects of using carbon dioxide for laparoscopic surgery in dogs. Vet Surg 1996;25:77–82.

14. Gilroy BA, Anson LW. Fatal air embolism during anesthesia for laparoscopy in a dog. J Am Vet Med Assoc 1987;190(5):552–4.

15. Staffieri F, Lacitignola L, De Siena R, et al. A case of spontaneous venous embolism with carbon dioxide during laparoscopic surgery in a pig. Vet Anaesth Analg 2007;34(1):63–6.

16. LeBlanc KA. General laparoscopic surgical complications. In: LeBlanc KA, editor. Management of laparoscopic surgical complications. New York: Marcel Dekker, Inc; 2004. p. 43–62.

17. McMahon AJ, Baxter JN, O'Dwyer PJ. Preventing complications of laparoscopy. Br J Surg 1993;80(12):1593–4.

18. Nickkholgh A, Barro-Bejarano M, Liang R, et al. Signs of reperfusion injury following CO_2 pneumoperitoneum: an in vivo microscopy study. Surg Endosc 2008;22(1):122–8.

19. Hanly EJ, Aurora AA, Shih SP, et al. Peritoneal acidosis mediates immunoprotection in laparoscopic surgery. Surgery 2007;142(3):357–64.

20. Bateman BG, Kolp LA, Hoeger K. Complications of laparoscopy – operative and diagnostic. Fertil Steril 1996;66(1):30–5.

21. Desmaizières LM, Martinot S, Lepage OM, et al. Complications associated with cannula insertion techniques used for laparoscopy in standing horses. Vet Surg 2003;32:501–6.

22. Kane MG, Krejs GJ. Complications of diagnostic laparoscopy in Dallas: a 7-year prospective study. Gastrointest Endosc 1984;30(4):237–40.
23. Heijnsdijk EA, de Visser H, Dankelman J, et al. Slip and damage properties of jaws of laparoscopic graspers. Surg Endosc 2004;18(6):974–9.
24. Bianchi PP, Rosati R, Bona S, et al. Laparoscopic surgery in rectal cancer: a prospective analysis of patient survival and outcomes. Dis Colon Rectum 2007;50(12):2047–53.
25. Kirchhoff P, Dincler S, Buchmann P. A multivariate analysis of potential risk factors for intra- and postoperative complications in 1316 elective laparoscopic colorectal procedures. Ann Surg 2008;248(2):259–65.
26. Feingold DL, Widmann WD, Calhoun SK, et al. Persistent post-laparoscopy pneumoperitoneum. Surg Endosc 2003;17(2):296–9.
27. Freeman LJ. Complications. In: Freeman LJ, editor. Veterinary endosurgery. St. Louis: Mosby, Inc; 1999. p. 92–102.
28. Brundell S, Ellis T, Dodd T, et al. Hematogenous spread as a mechanism for the generation of abdominal wound metastases following laparoscopy. Surg Endosc 2002;16(2):292–5.
29. Martinez J, Targarona EM, Balagué C, et al. Port site metastasis. An unresolved problem in laparoscopic surgery. A review. Int Surg 1995;80(4):315–21.
30. Paolucci V, Schaeff B, Schneider M, et al. Tumor seeding following laparoscopy: international survey. World J Surg 1999;23(10):989–95 [discussion: 996–7].
31. Lelievre L, Paterlini-Brechot P, Camatte S, et al. Effect of laparoscopy versus laparotomy on circulating tumor cells using isolation by size of epithelial tumor cells. Int J Gynecol Cancer 2004;14(2):229–33.
32. Tekkis PP, Senagore AJ, Delaney CP. Conversion rates in laparoscopic colorectal surgery. A predictive model with 1253 patients. Surg Endosc 2005;19:47–54.
33. Rotholtz, Laporte M, Pereyra L, et al. Predictive factors for conversion in laparoscopic colorectal surgery. Tech Coloproctol 2008;12:27–31.
34. Belizon A, Sardinha CT, Sher ME. Converted laparoscopic colectomy. What are the consequences? Surg Endosc 2006;20:947–51.
35. Schwandner O, Schiedeck TH, Bruch H. The role of conversion in laparoscopic colorectal surgery: do predictive factors exist? Surg Endosc 1999;13:151–6.
36. Shack C. Laparoscopic bowel surgery. Can Oper Room Nurs J 2007;25(2):6–8, 10–11, 13–14.
37. Pandya S, Murray JJ, Coller JA, et al. Laparoscopic colectomy. Indications for conversion to laparotomy. Arch Surg 1999;134(5):471–5.
38. Bowers SP, Hunter JG. Contraindications to laparoscopy. In: Whelan RL, Fleshman JW, Fowler DL, editors. The SAGES manual perioperative care in minimally invasive surgery. New York: Springer; 2006. p. 25–32.
39. Culp WT, Mayhew PD, Brown DC. A comparison of post-surgical activity in small dogs undergoing laparoscopic versus open ovariectomy. In: Proceedings of the 5th Annual Meeting of the Veterinary Endoscopy Society. Keystone; 2008. p. 4.
40. Hancock RB, Lanz OI, Waldron DR, et al. Comparison of postoperative pain after ovariohysterectomy by harmonic scalpel-assisted laparoscopy compared with median celiotomy and ligation in dogs. Vet Surg 2005;34:273–82.

Small Animal Exploratory Thoracoscopy

Chad Schmiedt, DVM

KEYWORDS

• Thoracoscopy • Dog • Cat • Veterinary • Endoscopy • Thorax

Exploratory thoracoscopy (ET) is used in veterinary surgery as a minimally invasive modality for the diagnosis and staging of intrathoracic disease. Although ET may be combined, either in the same or subsequent procedures, with some form of treatment, this article focuses entirely on the equipment and techniques for thoracoscopic exploration and biopsy.

Thoracoscopy has several advantages over more traditional, invasive thoracic exploration strategies. Compared with open thoracotomy, the superior illumination and magnification achieved with the thoracoscopic telescope allows for more accurate observation and interpretation of tissue morphology. Deep thoracic regions, which are challenging to evaluate in open procedures, may be more rapidly, accurately, and easily observed. Large tissue samples can be attained from specific lesions under direct observation, increasing the likelihood of accurate sample collection and diagnoses. Hemorrhage or air leakage resulting from a particular procedure can be identified immediately and corrected. Perhaps most importantly, ET is considerably less painful compared with open thoracotomy affording rapid surgical recovery.

ET has been compared with open thoracotomy in human and canine patients. In people, ET resulted in less acute postoperative pain,[1–3] faster recovery of pulmonary function,[1,3] less postoperative serum interleukin-6 concentration,[1] shorter general and intensive care hospitalization times,[4,5] shorter pleural drainage time,[4] and fewer complications.[4,5] However, ET also resulted in longer operative times[5] and did not offer any advantage in reduction of pain occurring more than 1 year after surgery.[2] In veterinary medicine, dogs undergoing thoracoscopic pericardectomy had reduced acute postoperative pain, blood glucose, and blood cortisol concentrations compared with dogs undergoing open thoracotomy.[6]

Department of Small Animal Medicine and Surgery, College of Veterinary Medicine, University of Georgia, 501 DW Brooks Drive, Athens, GA 30602, USA
E-mail address: cws@uga.edu

Vet Clin Small Anim 39 (2009) 953–964
doi:10.1016/j.cvsm.2009.05.007
0195-5616/09/$ – see front matter © 2009 Elsevier Inc. All rights reserved.

PREOPERATIVE DIAGNOSTICS AND INDICATIONS

Although less invasive than open thoracic exploration, ET is still an invasive procedure and should not be performed without a minimum database, including a complete blood count, serum biochemical analysis, urinalysis, and chest radiographs. Abdominal imagining with radiographs and ultrasound is frequently indicated to stage a neoplasm or rule out other abdominal disease. Radiographic or ultrasound-guided thoracocentesis may be indicated to provide initial diagnostic samples of pleural effusion. Patients with moderate or severe pleural effusion will benefit from therapeutic thoracocentesis to improve ventilation during anesthetic induction and patient preparation. Tracheobronchoscopy and bronchoalveolar lavage may provide diagnostic samples of bronchopulmonary infiltrates, as well as assist in planning thoracoscopic procedures. If one-lung intubation is planned, tracheobronchoscopy can be performed just before thoracoscopy in conjunction with placing bronchial blockers or verifying bronchial intubation.

Preoperative cross-sectional imaging is complimentary to ET. Preoperative thoracic CT or MRI allows the surgeon to plan patient positioning and portal location to maximize success and diagnostic yield of an ET procedure. Several CT-guided, percutaneous marking systems have been developed to preoperatively mark deep pulmonary lesions that may not be appreciated during ET, as they are well within pulmonary parenchyma.[7–10] These devices may be especially useful in larger veterinary patients with small pulmonary lesions, but their use has not been reported in this population.

There are several indications for ET. Diseases of the pleura may be definitively diagnosed using ET.[11] Thoracoscopically guided pleural biopsy provides tissue samples for histologic diagnosis of pleural effusions.[11] This can be particularly useful in patients with recurrent pleural effusion the cause of which is not apparent on cytologic examination or culture of the fluid. The cause of spontaneous pneumothorax may be diagnosed, localized, and staged using ET. The specific site of air leakage can be identified by partially filling the pleural space with saline and individually submerging lung lobes. When bubbles are seen coming from a lung lobe during positive pressure ventilation, a leakage site can be confirmed. All lung lobes should be evaluated, because patients may have multiple or bilateral lesions. Identification of multiple lesions should not deter surgical treatment, as prognosis with surgery is still good.[12,13]

Pyothorax is another potential indication for ET. In human pediatrics, early thoracoscopy for children with parapneumonic effusion or empyema significantly reduced hospitalization time and costs compared with the standard treatment using only a chest tube.[14,15] In addition to conformation of the diagnosis and searching for an etiology, thorough lavage of pleural space and debridement of fibrinous or necrotic material can also be performed. Occasionally, intrathoracic foreign bodies or abscessed lung lobes responsible for the pyothorax can be identified and removed. ET in patients with pyothorax can be challenging as adhesions, exudate, and fibrin will obscure and distort normal anatomy and limit working space. Although chylothorax is frequently diagnosed before surgery, the underlying cause may be determined with ET. Further, thoracic duct inspection and ligation, as well as a pericardectomy can be performed.[16,17] The diaphragm can also be evaluated it its entirety, and a diaphragmatic hernia can be diagnosed and repaired with thoracoscopy.[18]

Diagnostic biopsies of pleural or mediastinal mass lesions, enlarged lymph nodes, or pulmonary lesions may be obtained. Lung lobe torsion can be definitively diagnosed and treated. General pulmonary biopsies may be obtained in patients with diffuse interstitial lung disease. Pulmonary biopsies may be obtained completely intracorporally[19,20] or in conjunction with a keyhole thoracotomy[21] through thoracoscopic-assisted techniques. Confirmation of diagnosis or stage in patients with an intrathoracic neoplasm is an important application of ET in human medicine[22] and has a place in veterinary oncologic management. Similarly, staging of any intrathoracic mass may be performed and the likelihood of successful surgical resection evaluated.

Pericardial disease may be diagnosed and managed thoracoscopically.[23] The pericardium can be removed, submitted for biopsy, and the ventricular and atrial epicardium visually evaluated.

There are few contraindications for ET. Veterinary patients with traumatic thoracic injury will often respond to conservative management and do not require general anesthesia and thoracoscopic evaluation of pneumothorax or hemothorax; ET is contraindicated in most cases of acute trauma. ET may be performed in these patients if conservative management has failed or a diaphragmatic hernia is suspected and patients are judged as acceptable anesthetic candidates. As stated before, patients should not undergo this or other invasive procedures without appropriate preanesthetic diagnostic evaluations. Other contraindications relate to equipment and operator expertise. Anesthetic and thoracoscopic equipment should be functioning properly and appropriate for the patient size. Although select areas of the thorax may be evaluated with inappropriately sized instrumentation, a complete thoracic exploration is not possible. Likewise, practitioners should be familiar with basic thoracoscopic techniques before attempting ET.

ANESTHESIA AND POSITIONING

ET is performed under general anesthesia. Positive pressure, mechanical, or hand ventilation is necessary because an open pneumothorax is created. Expired carbon dioxide gas concentration and hemoglobin oxygen saturation should be monitored to evaluate ventilation. To increase the optical and working space, and improve visualization, especially for patients in lateral recumbency, one-lung intubation or mainstem bronchial blockade is effective. In healthy dogs on 100% oxygen there are minimal cardiopulmonary consequences to one-lung ventilation.[24] Several systems are available;[25] however, all are designed for people, and therefore, can be challenging to place in smaller veterinary patients. To prevent bronchial tube or blocker migration during patient preparation, bronchial intubation or blockade is most effectively established in the operating room after the patient has been positioned for surgery. Devices are positioned under tracheoscopic guidance. Diligent anesthetic monitoring is necessary during one-lung ventilation, as some bronchial blockers may migrate from the bronchus and cause acute tracheal obstruction. Malposition of lung isolation devices is a common complication in human ET anesthesia.[25]

In patients undergoing ET with standard tracheal intubation and ventilation, increasing ventilation rate and decreasing tidal volume is a strategy to increase working space while maintaining acceptable ventilation parameters. Constant communication with the anesthetist to maximize working space while maintaining patient safety is critical during ET. Often patient ventilation can be interrupted for brief periods of time to facilitate a particular observation or maneuver; similarly, during periods of surgical inactivity, normal or potentially more aggressive ventilation may be resumed.

Patients are positioned in dorsal, lateral, or sternal recumbency depending on the specific region of interest. The anesthetic and surgical team should always be prepared to convert to an open thoracotomy should the need arise. Therefore, a generous amount of skin is shaved, prepared, and draped for surgery to allow maximum flexibility of port placement and surgical options, should conversion to an open procedure become necessary. If the location of a lesion is not known precisely or if diffuse disease is suspected, dorsal recumbency is optimal, as it allows for the most complete evaluation of the two hemithoraces. The lateral or sternal position is used to evaluate structures in the lateral or dorsal thorax, respectively, and should be reserved for cases in which dorsal or lateral lesions are identified on preoperative diagnostic imagining. Complete and accurate thoracoscopic exploration is challenging, if not impossible, with the patient in sternal or lateral recumbency.

INSTRUMENTS

ET is performed with the standard rigid endoscopic instruments. A 0° or 30° telescope can be used. A 30° telescope offers more flexibility and requires less optical space to maneuver. These characteristics along with minimal image distortion make it a good choice for intrathoracic observation. The optimal telescope diameter and length will depend on the size of the patient. Large dogs will easily require a 10-mm diameter telescope, whereas in smaller dogs and cats, a 5-mm diameter telescope is appropriate. Larger telescopes will transmit a greater amount of light and provide a better field of view. A xenon light source should be used to illuminate the surgical field.

Intrathoracic insufflation is not advisable, so the instrument ports and cannulae should not create an airtight seal (see later discussion). Either screw-in or smooth ports can be used. Disposable ports are convenient as they can be cut to the desired length and sutured in place (**Fig. 1**). Although designed and marketed as disposable items, these ports can be gas sterilized and reused many times. Reusable metal laparoscopic ports can also be used, but tend to be too long and cumbersome. If laparoscopic ports are used, the valves should be removed to prevent the development of a tension pneumothorax. Establishing and maintaining a telescope port is recommended to prevent soiling the lens with blood and tissue as the telescope is removed and reintroduced into the pleural space. Instrument ports, however, are not absolutely necessary during ET. Although instrument ports may reduce tissue trauma from repeatedly withdrawing and inserting instruments, they may be forgone and instruments passed through small thoracotomies.

Retractors are often necessary to expose a lesion or area of interest. Outside of the chest, small or medium Gelpi retractors are often used in the skin, subcutis, and superficial musculature to provide tissue retraction of small thoracotomies. These

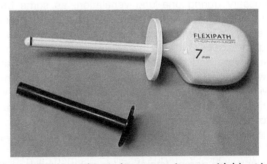

Fig.1. A smooth, disposable 7-mm Ethicon thoracoscopic port with blunt insertion obturator. The port is cut to the desired length and the introducer (above) is used to insert the port through the chest wall. The port is sutured to the skin to prevent displacement.

are also useful for retraction when performing thoracoscopic-assisted procedures. In the plural space, blunt and fan retractors are convenient for retracting lung lobes out of a working space or exposing hilar anatomy for examination. Blunt probes are commonly graduated in 1-cm increments to allow accurate thoracoscopic measurement. The fan retractor offers an adjustable broad surface to retract lung lobes and minimizes the risk of iatrogenic injury (**Fig. 2**). As with all endoscopic surgery, gravity offers the best retraction, so patient positioning is planned to facilitate gravitational retraction. Hydraulic surgery tables are available to facilitate perioperative manipulation of patient positioning.

Palpation can be accomplished using one of several instruments. The blunt probe also offers a safe and effective method of tissue palpation and is frequently used. Especially in smaller animals, traditional surgical instruments (forceps, hemostats, and so forth) may also be used as palpation devices or retractors; similarly, if a small thoracotomy is performed, digital palpation or retraction is also possible.

Lung tissue is usually manipulated with a blunt probe or endoscopic Babcock forceps. Care should be taken when manipulating lung tissue, particularly if there is no plan to remove tissue or if it is diffusely diseased. Minimal pressure, gentle handling, and use of an instrument with a broad grasping surface (**Fig. 3**) will minimize iatrogenic trauma. Conversely, tissue being removed, especially fibrous tissue such as the pericardium, is best manipulated with the so-called aggressive endoscopic graspers (**Fig. 4**). These graspers have traumatic interlocking teeth, which prevent tissue slippage when manipulating fibrous tissue.

One of the most useful instruments for biopsy is the cup biopsy forceps (**Fig. 5**). These are useful for pleural, mass, or lymph node biopsy. Endoscopic scissors can be used to bluntly and sharply dissect excisional or incisional biopsy specimens; some endoscopic scissors can be used with electrocautery to control hemorrhage from small vessels. However, because of the magnification and illumination afforded by the telescope, small vessels can often be identified and avoided to prevent hemorrhage. Generally, hemorrhage after biopsy is minimal and can usually be controlled with direct pressure. If available, endoscopic cautery or sealing devices may be used or procoagulant material may be placed over the area. Severe or uncontrollable hemorrhage is an indication for immediate conversion to an open thoracotomy.

Biopsy of lung tissue can be performed using several techniques. A pretied ligature can be used to encircle a small piece of lung tissue (**Fig. 6**). Tissue is then sharply cut distal to the ligature. A thin (~2–3 mm) cuff of tissue is left distal to the ligature to prevent slippage of the ligature. This technique is restricted to small lesions on the margin of a lung lobe. Should larger biopsy samples be required, an endoscopic gastrointestinal anastomosis stapling and cutting device (Endo-GIA, Coviden, Mansfield, MA) can be used to perform a partial or complete lobectomy. These stapling and cutting devices

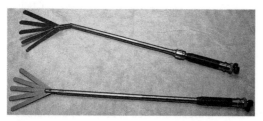

Fig. 2. Ten-millimeter fan retractors provide an adjustable, broad retraction instrument for thorascopic exploration.

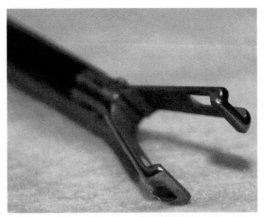

Fig. 3. The broad, atraumatic, grasping surface of endoscopic Babcock forceps is designed to prevent iatrogenic trauma to delicate tissue.

are available in a variety of lengths and staple sizes that attach to a reusable hand piece. To prevent leakage, the smallest possible staple size should be employed. A more thorough description of lung lobectomy is available in another article.

Pulmonary biopsies can also be obtained using endoscopic instruments, which deliver different forms of energy. An endoscopic bipolar sealing device (Ligasure, Tyco Healthcare Group, Boulder, Colorado) can be used to obtain a lung biopsy. In healthy pigs, the bipolar sealing device created an air seal as strong as a stapled lung biopsy site and normal lung.[26] In human patients with lung disease who are undergoing a lung biopsy, the bipolar sealing device also appeared to perform well.

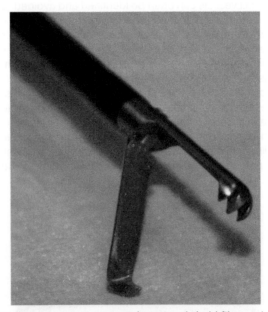

Fig. 4. Aggressive endoscopic graspers are used to securely hold fibrous tissue or tissue being removed. These graspers should not be used on delicate tissue, especially if being left in the patient.

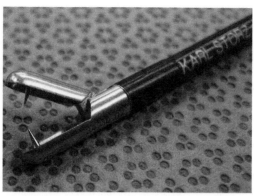

Fig. 5. Endoscopic cup biopsy forceps are useful for biopsy of pleura, lymph node, or masses. Spikes within the cup prevent tissue slippage while the instrument is being closed.

Out of 36 patients, none experienced blood leakage and two experienced prolonged (>7 days) air leakage.[27] Recently, this instrument has been reported to be successful for biopsy of lung tissue in heaves-affected horses. Eighteen out of 28 of these horses developed postoperative pneumothorax, which resolved in all but one.[28]

Alternatively, use of an ultrasonic cutting and coagulation device (Harmonic Scalpel, Ethicon Endo-Surgery Inc., Cincinnati, Ohio) has been described for obtaining lung biopsies. In rabbits, the harmonic scalpel functioned well and created an air seal resistant to approximately 32.5 cmH$_2$O.[29] Although leakage pressure was not evaluated, the harmonic scalpel also resulted in no complications when used to obtain lung biopsies in healthy research dogs.[30] However, clinical use of the harmonic scalpel in human patients has met with mixed reviews due to a higher than desirable incidence of postbiopsy air leakage.[31,32] Indeed, the positive results presented here for endoscopic energy delivery devices should be interpreted with caution, as the maximal bronchial diameter that either instrument is capable of sealing is unknown, and their efficacy and complications have not been reported in small animal patients. Regardless of the technique employed to obtain a lung biopsy, one should verify the biopsy is not leaking with the submersion technique before closure.

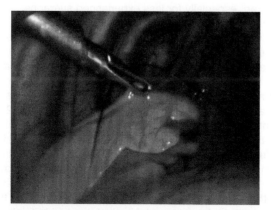

Fig. 6. The distal portion of a lung lobe is being retracted with endoscopic Babcock forceps. A pretied ligature loop is being placed around the lung lobe. The suture will be tightened using an endoscopic knot pusher and the lung distal to the ligature will be excised.

A suction-irrigation device is useful for pleural lavage. This tool also provides a method of instilling and removing saline to check lung lobes for air leakage and lavage the plural space. A single unit endoscopic suction-irrigation device is convenient; as it abrogates the need for switching irrigation and suction instruments. Peristaltic pumps are available to facilitate saline delivery. A 1- or 5-L bag of saline elevated over the patient in a pressurized bag offers a less expensive alternative.

TECHNIQUES

Pneumothorax is essential for ET as it causes the lung lobes to fall away from the chest wall, establishing an optical and working space. Unlike laparoscopy, intrathoracic insufflation is not necessary or desirable during almost all ET procedures. Intrathoracic insufflation, even at low pressures (3–5 mmHg), may result in a reduction of cardiac output and, therefore, should be used with caution and only when sufficient monitoring equipment and expertise are available and a clear indication exists.[33] Other than intrathoracic insufflation, pneumothorax can be established using one of two alternative methods.[34] The first technique is one-lung ventilation, discussed earlier, and is useful for establishing an optical and working space. Alternating one-lung ventilation may be a strategy for maximizing working space in procedures that require work in both hemithoraces.[35] The second technique, used frequently when procedures are limited to ET, is a simple semi-open pneumothorax with standard endotracheal intubation. This method is the simplest for establishing a working space. The technique seems most effective when performing thoracoscopy with the patient in dorsal recumbency.

A pneumothorax is created to facilitate the insertion of the telescope cannula. Blunt and sharp techniques are described.[34] For sharp insertion, a pneumothorax is first created by percutaneously inserting a Veres needle into the pleural space. The Veres needle allows air to enter the thorax. Once enough air has entered the pleural space to allow the lungs to fall away from the chest wall, a cannula with a sharp trochar is inserted. Alternatively, a blunt technique is used. The skin is incised and blunt dissection is used to gain access to the chest cavity. Once a tract has been created with blunt dissection, a cannula is inserted with a blunt trochar. A small pneumothorax will usually result from the blunt dissection and develop rapidly after the obturator is removed and the cannula is open to the atmosphere. The blunt technique is most frequently used as it is easy, rapid, and affords less risk of iatrogenic trauma. This technique is preferred, especially for less experienced surgeons.

Telescope portals are established in a paraxiphoid or intercostal location. The paraxiphoid position is used for ET performed in dorsal recumbency. The xiphoid cartilage is palpated and a small skin incision is made just lateral to the cartilage. Kelly or Carmalt hemostats are used to create a cranially, and slightly dorsally, directed tunnel into the caudal ventral most aspect of the thoracic cavity. A screw-in or smooth port can then be placed using a blunt trochar. If lateral patient positioning is used, an intercostal telescope portal can be established in a similar manner. A small (~2 cm) skin incision is made and blunt dissection with hemostats or Metzenbaum scissors is used to establish a tract through the subcutaneous tissue and intercostal musculature. A cannula with a blunt obturator is then inserted. The lateral port is generally placed slightly away from the lesion to increase the field of view and allow for instrument triangulation.

After a pneumothorax is established and the telescope is inserted the thorax can be explored. If a paraxiphoid telescope portal is used, the caudo-ventral mediastinum is observed on midline effectively equally dividing the two hemithoraces. The caudo-ventral mediastinum will have to be broken down to effectively evaluate the entire intrathoracic space. In normal dogs and cats the caudo-ventral mediastinum is a thin, opaque membrane, which can be easily perforated with a blunt dissection instrument or with the scope itself. In patients with chronic pleural disease, this membrane can be thick, tough, and more vascular, and may require careful dissection and hemostasis.

Exploration should be thorough and systematic. The diaphragm, mediastinum, chest wall, lung lobes, pericardium, lymph nodes, great vessels, esophagus, and epicardium can be observed. A complete thoracic exploration should be performed before performing biopsies or other procedures. Establishment of at least one working portal is often required to provide retraction and facilitate exploration. An exception to performing a complete exploration before any procedure may be in cases whereby pathology obscures anatomy and removal or drainage is required to complete exploration. For example, little visual and working space is available in dogs with severe chronic pericardial effusion; however, once the effusion is drained, much more space is available and exploration can be completed.

At least one instrument port is usually needed for a retraction, palpation, or biopsy instrument. The optimal location for this instrument port is chosen and a blunt or sharp insertion technique is used. If a thoracoscopic-assisted procedure is planned, one of the instrument ports should be located in a position that can be easily converted into a mini-thoracotomy to facilitate exteriorization of tissue. While establishing instrument ports, it is prudent to observe the site intrathoracically with the telescope to prevent iatrogenic trauma and facilitate accurate port placement. Instrument ports should be placed as needed in strategically appropriate positions. A surgeon should not feel limited in the number of instrument portals to create; should the task at hand require additional portals, additional portal should be added. To facilitate triangulation of the telescope, instrument, and the tissue of interest, several principles should be followed.[34]

Intrathoracic location of planned portals should be confirmed by viewing the plural surface of the chest wall while palpating the skin with a finger or instrument. The resulting indention observed in the chest wall confirms the eventual location of the instrument port. This exercise is important and should be repeated with each new port, as port position is not always apparent based on extrathoracic reckoning. Instrument portals should be placed far enough apart to not interfere with each other or the telescope. Working portals that are close together, or close to the telescope, often do not add strategic value and frequently interfere with each other or with the telescope. A baseball field analogy is frequently used. If a specific tissue or lesion is home base, the relative telescope position should be around second base. First and third base should be the relative positions of instrument ports. Instrument ports can also be appropriately added in planes above and below the telescope. To finish the analogy, the video monitor is ideally placed behind the home plate to be in the direct line of site of the surgeon.

The variability of available instruments and tissue morphology preclude an exhaustive description of biopsy techniques. Biopsies can be obtained with several different instruments and techniques. It is always worth the time and effort to obtain multiple biopsies, especially if small amounts of tissue are being taken or gross pathology is not present. Prior to biopsy, palpation can be accomplished with a blunt probe, a finger, or other instrument. Thoracoscopic-guided aspiration of unknown structures or lesions with spinal needles may be useful to determine the safest biopsy technique. An excellent labeled atlas of normal and abnormal intrathoracic tissue morphology as observed with a thoracoscope has been published and is recommended for new endoscopists.[34]

After ET is completed, a chest tube is placed to remove air or residual fluid from the pleural space. Placement of the chest tube can be confirmed by observation through the telescope. Closure of ports should be done depending on their size. If a significant defect in the chest wall exists, circumcostal sutures may be necessary; however, this is frequently not the case. One or two interrupted sutures in the intercostal musculature are necessary in the telescope portals and the skin and subcutaneous tissue are closed routinely.

Complications of ET are predictable. Anesthetic complications relating to hypoventilation with resulting hypoxemia and hypercarbia may result if ventilation is not adequately or accurately monitored. Similarly, acute, fatal tracheal obstruction is possible if bronchial blocking devices migrate. Blood or air leakage is possible when biopsies are performed; consequently, biopsied tissues should be critically evaluated for leakage afterward. Portal metastasis has been reported in a dog following thoracoscopic biopsy of mesothelioma and should be included as a risk if a neoplasm is suspected and a biopsy is performed.[36]

REFERENCES

1. Nagahiro I, Andou A, Aoe M, et al. Pulmonary function, postoperative pain, and serum cytokine level after lobectomy: a comparison of VATS and conventional procedure. Ann Thorac Surg 2001;72(2):362–5.
2. Landreneau RJ, Mack MJ, Hazelrigg SR, et al. Prevalence of chronic pain after pulmonary resection by thoracotomy or video-assisted thoracic surgery. J Thorac Cardiovasc Surg 1994;107(4):1079–85 [discussion: 1085–76].
3. Landreneau RJ, Hazelrigg SR, Mack MJ, et al. Postoperative pain-related morbidity: video-assisted thoracic surgery versus thoracotomy. Ann Thorac Surg 1993;56(6):1285–9.
4. Weatherford DA, Stephenson JE, Taylor SM, et al. Thoracoscopy versus thoracotomy: indications and advantages. Am Surg 1995;61(1):83–6.
5. Ferson PF, Landreneau RJ, Dowling RD, et al. Comparison of open versus thoracoscopic lung biopsy for diffuse infiltrative pulmonary disease. J Thorac Cardiovasc Surg 1993;106(2):194–9.
6. Walsh PJ, Remedios AM, Ferguson JF, et al. Thoracoscopic versus open partial pericardectomy in dogs: comparison of postoperative pain and morbidity. Vet Surg 1999;28(6):472–9.
7. Dendo S, Kanazawa S, Ando A, et al. Preoperative localization of small pulmonary lesions with a short hook wire and suture system: experience with 168 procedures. Radiology 2002;225(2):511–8.
8. Koyama H, Noma S, Tamaki Y, et al. CT localisation of small pulmonary nodules prior to thorascopic resection: evaluation of a point marker system. Eur J Radiol 2008;65(3):468–72.
9. Mack MJ, Gordon MJ, Postma TW, et al. Percutaneous localization of pulmonary nodules for thoracoscopic lung resection. Ann Thorac Surg 1992;53(6):1123–4.
10. Thaete FL, Peterson MS, Plunkett MB, et al. Computed tomography-guided wire localization of pulmonary lesions before thoracoscopic resection: results in 101 cases. J Thorac Imaging 1999;14(2):90–8.
11. Kovak JR, Ludwig LL, Bergman PJ, et al. Use of thoracoscopy to determine the etiology of pleural effusion in dogs and cats: 18 cases (1998–2001). J Am Vet Med Assoc 2002;221(7):990–4.
12. Lipscomb VJ, Hardie RJ, Dubielzig RR. Spontaneous pneumothorax caused by pulmonary blebs and bullae in 12 dogs. J Am Anim Hosp Assoc 2003;39(5): 435–45.

13. Puerto DA, Brockman DJ, Lindquist C, et al. Surgical and nonsurgical management of and selected risk factors for spontaneous pneumothorax in dogs: 64 cases (1986–1999). J Am Vet Med Assoc 2002;220(11):1670–4.
14. Aziz A, Healey JM, Qureshi F, et al. Comparative analysis of chest tube thoracostomy and video-assisted thoracoscopic surgery in empyema and parapneumonic effusion associated with pneumonia in children. Surg Infect (Larchmt) 2008;9(3):317–23.
15. Gates RL, Caniano DA, Hayes JR, et al. Does VATS provide optimal treatment of empyema in children? A systematic review. J Pediatr Surg 2004;39(3):381–6.
16. Radlinsky MG, Mason DE, Biller DS, et al. Thoracoscopic visualization and ligation of the thoracic duct in dogs. Vet Surg 2002;31(2):138–46.
17. Enwiller TM, Radlinsky MG, Mason DE, et al. Popliteal and mesenteric lymph node injection with methylene blue for coloration of the thoracic duct in dogs. Vet Surg 2003;32(4):359–64.
18. Adamiak Z, Holak P, Szalecki P. Thoracoscopic treatment of the diaphragmatic hernia in dog – case report. Medycyna Weterynaryjna 2008;64(2):210–2.
19. Faunt KK, Jones BD, Turk JR, et al. Evaluation of biopsy specimens obtained during thoracoscopy from lungs of clinically normal dogs. Am J Vet Res 1998; 59(11):1499–502.
20. Boutin C, Viallat JR, Cargnino P, et al. Thoracoscopic lung biopsy. Experimental and clinical preliminary study. Chest 1982;82(1):44–8.
21. Norris CR, Griffey SM, Walsh P. Use of keyhole lung biopsy for diagnosis of interstitial lung diseases in dogs and cats: 13 cases (1998–2001). J Am Vet Med Assoc 2002;221(10):1453–9.
22. Detterbeck FC, DeCamp MM Jr, Kohman LJ, et al. Invasive staging: the guidelines. Chest 2003;123(90010):167S–75S.
23. Jackson J, Richter KP, Launer DP. Thoracoscopic partial pericardiectomy in 13 dogs. J Vet Intern Med 1999;13(6):529–33.
24. Cantwell SL, Duke T, Walsh PJ, et al. One-lung versus two-lung ventilation in the closed-chest anesthetized dog: a comparison of cardiopulmonary parameters. Vet Surg 2000;29(4):365–73.
25. Campos JH. Which device should be considered the best for lung isolation: double-lumen endotracheal tube versus bronchial blockers. Curr Opin Anaesthesiol 2007;20(1):27–31.
26. Tirabassi MV, Banever GT, Tashjian DB, et al. Quantitation of lung sealing in the survival swine model. J Pediatr Surg 2004;39(3):387–90.
27. Santini M, Vicidomini G, Baldi A, et al. Use of an electrothermal bipolar tissue sealing system in lung surgery. Eur J Cardiothorac Surg 2006;29(2):226–30.
28. Relave F DF, Leclere M, Alexander K, et al. Evaluation of a bipolar sealing tissue sealing system to performed thorascopic lung biopsy in heaves affected horses. American College of Veterinary Surgeons Veterinary Symposium. vol. 37. San Diego (CA): Wilie; 2008. p. E9.
29. Samancilar O, Cakan A, Cetin Y, et al. Comparison of the harmonic scalpel and the ultrasonic surgical aspirator in subsegmental lung resections: an experimental study. Thorac Cardiovasc Surg 2007;55(8):509–11.
30. Molnar TF, Szanto Z, Laszlo T, et al. Cutting lung parenchyma using the harmonic scalpel – an animal experiment. Eur J Cardiothorac Surg 2004;26(6):1192–5.
31. Molnar TF, Benko I, Szanto Z, et al. Lung biopsy using harmonic scalpel: a randomised single institute study. Eur J Cardiothorac Surg 2005;28(4):604–6.
32. Molnar TF, Benko I, Szanto Z, et al. Complications after ultrasonic lung parenchyma biopsy: a strong note for caution. Surg Endosc 2008;22(3):679–82.

33. Daly CM, Swalec-Tobias K, Tobias AH, et al. Cardiopulmonary effects of intrathoracic insufflation in dogs. J Am Anim Hosp Assoc 2002;38(6):515–20.
34. McCarthy TC, Monnet E. Diagnostic and operative thoracoscopy. In: McCarthy TC, editor. Veterinary endoscopy. St. Louis (MO): Elsevier Saunders; 2005. p. 229–78.
35. Russell K, MP, Sorrell-Raschi L. Thoracoscopic subphrenic pericardectomy using double lumen endobronchial intubation for alternating one lung ventilation. Article presented at: American College of Veterinary Surgeons Veterinary Symposium. San Diego (CA), October 23-25, 2008.
36. Brisson BA, Reggeti F, Bienzle D. Portal site metastasis of invasive mesothelioma after diagnostic thoracoscopy in a dog. J Am Vet Med Assoc 2006;229(6):980–3.

Interventional Thoracoscopy in Small Animals

Eric Monnet, DVM, PhD, FAHA

KEYWORDS

- Minimally invasive surgery • Thoracic surgery • Dog
- Cat • Techniques

Thoracoscopy is a minimally invasive technique for viewing the internal structures of the thoracic cavity. The procedure uses a rigid telescope placed through a portal positioned in the thoracic wall to examine the contents of the pleural cavity. Once the telescope is in place, either biopsy forceps or an assortment of surgical instruments can be introduced into the thoracic cavity through adjacent portals in the thoracic wall to perform various diagnostic or surgical procedures. The minimal invasiveness of the procedure, the rapid patient recovery, and the diagnostic accuracy make thoracoscopy an ideal technique compared with other more invasive procedures.

Despite the advent of newer laboratory tests, imaging techniques, and ultrasound-directed fine needle biopsy or aspiration, thoracoscopy remains a valuable tool when appropriately applied in a diagnostic plan. Thoracoscopy may also provide accurate and definitive diagnostic and staging information that would otherwise be obtained through an open thoracotomy.[1] Small animal thoracoscopy has not only developed into a diagnostic tool but also has progressed to a means for minimally invasive surgical procedures.

Interventional thoracoscopy is an emerging surgical technique in veterinary surgery used to perform pericardial window, subtotal pericardiectomy, or lung lobectomy to correct vascular ring anomalies, to ligate patent ductus arteriosus and the thoracic duct, and to aid in the treatment of pyothorax.[1–10] Most procedures are performed under thoracoscopy, and some procedures can be thoracoscopically assisted.

PERICARDIAL WINDOW AND SUBTOTAL PERICARDIECTOMY

Creation of a window in the pericardium or a subtotal pericardiectomy establishes permanent drainage for patients with pericardial effusion.[4,5,7] This technique is performed effectively with greatly reduced operative trauma and postoperative pain.[7] Indications for permanent pericardial drainage include neoplastic effusion, hemorrhage from neoplastic masses, inflammatory disease, and idiopathic effusion. This

Department of Clinical Sciences, Colorado State University, 300 W Drake Road, Fort Collins, CO 80523, USA
E-mail address: eric.monnet@colostate.edu

Vet Clin Small Anim 39 (2009) 965–975
doi:10.1016/j.cvsm.2009.05.005
0195-5616/09/$ – see front matter © 2009 Elsevier Inc. All rights reserved.

vetsmall.theclinics.com

procedure prevents cardiac tamponade by allowing drainage of pericardial fluid into the pleural space. This technique dramatically improves quality of life in cases of neoplasia. It allows rapid recovery and return of the patient to the owner's care.

Approach

The patient is placed in dorsal recumbency or in left lateral recumbency to perform a pericardial window.[4,5,7] One-lung ventilation is not required, even for a subtotal pericardiectomy.[4]

Transdiaphragmatic approach

If the patient is placed in dorsal recumbency, a para-xiphoid, transdiaphragmatic approach is used to place the endoscope. Then there are two options for placing operative portals.

The easiest technique is to place one portal on the right and one on the left side of the thoracic cavity. Triangulation is respected with this approach, making the surgery easier. The mediastinum has to be dissected to visualize both sides of the thoracic cavity. The operative portals are placed in the left and right ninth to tenth intercostal spaces. The surgeon can stand on either side of the patient. Tilting the patient slightly to the left (10°–15°) facilitates visualization and manipulation. After all portals are in place, the ventral mediastinum is incised from the sternum to remove it from the surgical field. Scissors are used with electrosurgical assistance for hemostasis. Inadequate control of bleeding from the mediastinal vessels interferes with the procedure by allowing blood contamination of the telescope tip, which obscures visualization. The telescope operator stands at the foot of the patient or across the patient from the surgeon.

The other technique is to place both instrument portals on the right side. With this approach, the triangulation technique is not respected, but the mediastinum does not have to be dissected. The operative portals are in the right sixth or seventh intercostal space and in the right ninth or tenth intercostal space. The surgeon stands on the right side of the patient, and the telescope operator stands at the foot of the patient or across the patient from the surgeon.

Intercostal approach

As an alternative, an intercostal approach can be performed. This approach allows for a better visualization of the right atrial appendage and aortic root to evaluate for the presence of a heart base tumor.

The patient is placed in left lateral recumbency, and the camera portal is placed in the ventral third of the sixth or seventh intercostal space. Two instrument portals are then placed in the fourth intercostal and the eighth intercostal spaces. A pericardial window is then performed on the right side of the pericardium. The phrenic nerve must be identified before incising the pericardium.

Surgical Technique

Pericardial window

The technique performed through a transdiaphragmatic or an intercostal approach is similar.[5]

First, explore the cranial mediastinum for lymph-node enlargement, and biopsy any abnormality identified. Biopsy of the lymph node may reveal the diagnosis of mesothelioma of the pericardium, which might not be diagnosed on the pericardial sample submitted for histology.

A site is selected for the pericardial window on the cranial surface of the heart toward the apex. The apex of the heart falls dorsally when pneumothorax is established with the patient in dorsal recumbency, presenting the cranial surface of the heart to the surgeon rather than the apex, which would be seen without the pneumothorax present. Babcock forceps or aggressive grasping forceps with teeth are used to grasp and elevate a fold of pericardium, and Metzenbaum scissors are used to incise the fold for initial penetration of the pericardium (**Fig. 1**). The graspers are repositioned to lift 1 margin of the initial pericardial incision. Remove with suction any excess pericardial fluid that has not been previously evacuated and that interferes with visualization. Extend the pericardial incision with electrocautery or a vessel sealant device (Ligasure, Valley Lab, Boulder, Colorado) to remove a segment of pericardium, taking care not to damage the phrenic nerves, heart, lungs, or great vessels.

There are no scientific data to define how much pericardium to remove. The portion removed needs to be large enough to prevent closure of the defect by the healing process and small enough to preclude herniation of the heart through the window. A window 4 × 4 cm has been recommended.[5] The pericardial sample is extracted from the thoracic cavity through one of the operative portals and is inspected for size. Samples are submitted for histopathology and culture.

After completion of the pericardial window, pericardioscopy can be performed to visualize the inside of the pericardium for signs of mesothelioma and to evaluate the right atrial appendage and the aortic root (**Fig. 2**). Usually an angle endoscope helps to inspect the aortic root.

Any residual pericardial and/or pleural fluid is removed with suction, and the cavities are irrigated with saline. Operative portal cannulas are removed, and the port sites apposed in layers to achieve an airtight closure. A thoracostomy tube is placed in routine fashion. Placement of the tube can be visualized and controlled with the endoscope.

Subtotal pericardiectomy

The primary indication for subtotal pericardiectomy is constrictive pericarditis. Subtotal pericardiectomy may also be indicated for infectious processes or neoplasia involving an extensive area of the pericardium. The dissection for subtotal pericardiectomy is much more difficult than for creating a pericardial window. Place the patient in dorsal recumbency for a transdiaphragmatic approach.[4] Identify the phrenic nerves (**Fig. 3**). The pericardium is incised ventral to the phrenic nerves. Start the pericardial excision in the same manner as for creating a pericardial window, but extend the

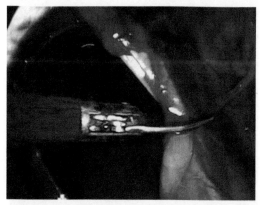

Fig. 1. Pericardium is incised with Metzembaum scissors. Pericardial fluid is still present in the pericardial sac.

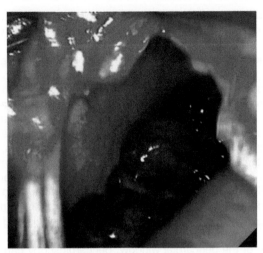

Fig. 2. A right atrial tumor visualized in the pericardial sac.

pericardial incision as far cranially and dorsally as possible and circumferentially in each direction. Electrosurgical assistance is used as needed for hemostasis. Portal closure, chest tube placement, and postoperative management are the same as for a pericardial window.

LUNG LOBECTOMY

Partial and complete lung lobectomy are possible under thoracoscopy for the excision of small peripheral lesions or the resection of primary lung tumors.[8]

Partial Lung Lobectomy

Lung biopsy for chronic lung disease, excision of lung masses, lung abscesses, emphysematous bullae, or any other localized disease process in the peripheral

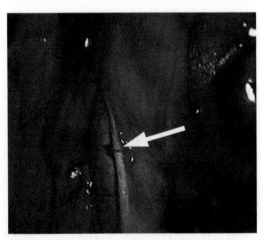

Fig. 3. Phrenic nerve (*arrow*) along the caudal vena cava and the pericardium.

portions of the lung lobes can be performed quickly and effectively with a minimally invasive technique.[3,8,11]

Approach

Portal placement for partial lung lobectomy is dictated by the location of the lung to be removed. Dorsal recumbency and para-xiphoid telescope portal allow examination of both sides of the chest for cases in which the side of the pathology cannot be determined (eg, spontaneous pneumothorax). Lateral recumbency provides greater unilateral access and is the preferred position if the involved side can be determined preoperatively with radiographs, ultrasound, or CT. The telescope and operative portals are inserted using appropriate triangulation to access the involved pathology.

An alternative procedure is to perform a thoracoscopally assisted partial lung lobectomy. The technique is performed in lateral recumbency with an intercostal approach. The portion of lung to be resected is exteriorized, and the resection is completed outside the thoracic cavity.

Surgical technique

For peripheral lesions less than 2 cm in diameter, a loop ligature technique can be used. The tip of the lobe to be removed is positioned through a pretied loop ligature, which is then tightened. The ligated portion of the lung is transected and removed. This technique is possible only if the suture can be placed no more than 3 cm from the edge of the lung. Larger or more central lesions require an endoscopic stapling device for occlusion and transection of the portion of the lobe to be removed.

When performing partial lung lobectomy with an endoscopic stapler (EndoGIA, AutoSuture, Mansfield, Massachusetts), place the endoscopic stapler through an additional portal to provide optimal alignment for application of the stapler. After transection of the lung lobe, the excised portion is removed by enlarging one of the portals to allow passage of the tissue. An endoscopic tissue pouch can be used to facilitate tissue removal. Observe the transected lung margin for air leakage or hemorrhage before removing the telescope from the chest. Place a thoracostomy tube at a site away from all portals, remove the operative and telescope cannulas, and close the port sites.

When performing a thoracoscopically assisted lung lobectomy, a cannula hole is enlarged to exteriorize and resect the abnormal portion of lung. The lung resection is then performed outside the thoracic cavity with either staples or hand suturing (**Fig. 4**).

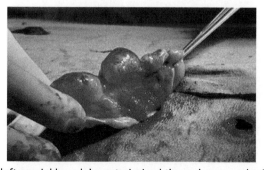

Fig. 4. Bullae on a left cranial lung lobe exteriorized through a cannula site during a thoracoscopic-assisted partial lung lobectomy.

Complete Lung Lobectomy

Approach

Lung lobes with small masses located away from the pulmonary hilus can be removed with minimally invasive surgery. Large masses impair visualization of the hilus of the lung and make manipulation of the lung difficult.[8,11] Lateral recumbency with intercostal portal placement is the preferred technique for complete lung lobectomy. One-lung ventilation is recommended to increase the amount of space available in the thoracic cavity to manipulate the instruments and the lung mass.[8,11,12] One-lung ventilation is induced after the patient has been positioned on the operating table to avoid dislodging the bronchial obturator. Place the patient in an oblique position to improve the exposure of the dorsal part of the pulmonary hilus.

Place a telescope portal and two operative portals with triangulation, and prepare the hilus of the lung lobe to be removed with sharp dissection. A fourth portal is required for the placement of the stapling equipment.

Surgical technique

Pulmonary artery, vein, and bronchi are not isolated at the hilus for minimally invasive lung lobectomy (**Fig. 5**). For caudal lung lobes, the pulmonary ligament is divided to free the lung lobe for manipulation.[8]

Place a 45 to 65 mm–long EndoGIA stapling cartridge with 3.5 mm staples across the hilus of the lobe. The staple line is placed perpendicular to the hilus to maximize the length of the staple line (**Fig. 6**). It is important to ensure that no structures other than the hilus of the lung are in the stapler equipment before firing the stapler. An angle endoscope makes this step easier. The stapling cartridge must be long enough to include the entire hilus of the lung to be removed. A 65 mm–long cartridge is most commonly used. Place the resected lung lobe in a retrieval or specimen bag to prevent seeding of the thoracic wall. Enlarge a cannula hole to retrieve the lung lobe in the retrieval bag. Enlarged hilar lymph nodes should be biopsied or removed. If a lymph node is sampled, use a combination of sharp and blunt dissection to isolate the lymph

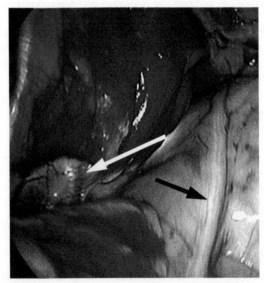

Fig. 5. Hilus of the lung (*white arrow*) and phrenic nerve (*black arrow*) on the pericardium.

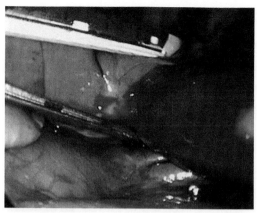

Fig. 6. A stapling device applied to the hilus of the lung for lobectomy.

node. Electrosurgical assistance and clip application can be used for hemostasis. Before removal of the telescope, observe the hilus for air leakage or hemorrhage. Place a thoracostomy tube at a site away from all portals, remove the operative and telescope portals, and close the port sites.

CORRECTION OF PERSISTENT RIGHT AORTIC ARCH

Correction of esophageal compression by a ligamentum arteriosum associated with a persistent right aortic arch (PRAA) is possible in dogs.[9]

Approach

Place the patient in right lateral recumbency, and place telescope and operative portals in the left sixth or seventh intercostal space. Place the telescope portal at the junction of the dorsal and middle third of the intercostal space. Place the operative portals on either side of the telescope portal. A fourth portal might be required to introduce a retractor for the left cranial lung lobe. This portal is placed in the sixth or seventh intercostal space at the level of the costochondral junction to retract the lobe caudally.

Surgical Technique

A pediatric set of instruments (2.7 mm) is recommended for this surgery. The first step of the procedure is to localize the ligamentum arteriosum. Move the cranial lung lobe away from the cranial mediastinum. Then place a stomach tube in the esophagus to improve visualization of the ligamentum arteriosum. Use a palpation probe to localize the ligamentum arteriosum.

Dissect the ligamentum arteriosum with sharp and blunt dissection to isolate it from the pleura and esophagus (**Fig. 7**). Passing a stomach tube or an endoscope facilitates identification of the esophagus during dissection. Because some ligamentum arteriosum are patent at the time of surgery, it is recommended to either place vascular clips or use a vessel sealant device on the ligamentum arteriosum (**Fig. 8**), which is then transected between the clips or the seals. Dissect any remaining fibers from the esophagus (**Fig. 9**). A balloon dilation catheter can be used to further dilate the esophagus under thoracoscopic visualization. If the esophagus is not totally free, more fibers

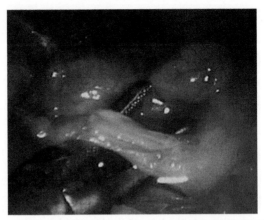

Fig. 7. The ligamentum arteriosum has been dissected with a curved hemostat.

have to be dissected. Place a thoracostomy tube and close the port sites. Postoperative dietary management is the same as for open surgical PRAA correction.

LIGATION OF THORACIC DUCT

Management of chylothorax by thoracic duct occlusion is far easier with minimally invasive technique than with an open surgical approach.[10,13] Magnification produced by the telescope and video system greatly enhances visualization of the thoracic ducts, and instrumentation designed for minimally invasive surgery facilitates manipulation of structures deep in the chest.

Approach

Place the patient in sternal recumbency to expose the dorsal aspect of the thoracic cavity. The weight of the lung provides enough retraction to visualize the target structures.[10]

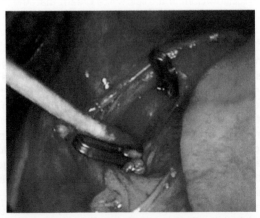

Fig. 8. Two vascular clips have been applied on the ligamentum arteriosum before transection.

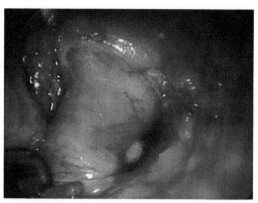

Fig. 9. Fibers have been completely dissected from the esophagus. The esophagus is dilated with a balloon. The clips are hiding on either side of the esophagus.

Place the telescope portal in the eighth intercostal space at the dorsoventral midpoint of the intercostal space in the right side. Place operative portals between the telescope portal and the dorsal end of the ribs in the ninth and tenth intercostal spaces.

Methylene blue injection in the popliteal lymph node, a mesenteric lymph node, or in the cysterna chyle has been recommended to improve visualization of the thoracic duct.[13]

Surgical Technique

Use a grasping forceps and scissors connected to an electrocautery unit to dissect the dorsal part of the caudal mediastinum and identify the thoracic duct. Dissection has to be performed until the left hemithorax is entered. Ligate each branch of the thoracic duct with one or two vascular clips.

Efficacy of thoracic duct occlusion for management of chylothorax is questionable and controversial. If this method of treatment is elected or indicated, the substantially reduced trauma associated with a thoracoscopic approach is of great benefit to the patient.

LIGATION OF PATENT DUCTUS ARTERIOSUS

Ligation of patent ductus arteriosus is a routine procedure in pediatric cardiac surgery. Patent ductus arteriosus has been performed with success on five dogs under thoracoscopy or under thoracoscopic-assisted visualization.[2]

Approach

Place the patient in right lateral recumbency, and place portals in the middle and dorsal aspects of the intercostal space.[2]

If thoracoscopic-assisted visualization is used, a thoracoscopic portal is placed in the fifth intercostal space.

If a thoracoscopic ligation is performed, the thoracoscopic portal is placed in the fourth or third intercostal space, midway between the sternum and the dorsal spinal process. Two other portals are placed in the fifth intercostal space. One is placed half way between the sternum and the dorsal spinal process, the other is placed in the dorsal third of the intercostal space.[2]

Surgical Techniques

A 2 to 3 cm intercostal thoracotomy is performed in the fifth intercostal space for the thoracoscopic-assisted technique. Dissection of the patent ductus arteriosus is conducted as with thoracotomy through the mini-thoracotomy under thoracoscopic visualization.

For the thoracoscopic technique, introduce a retractor in the ventral portal to retract the left cranial lung lobe. Use a dissecting hook connected to electrocautery in the most dorsal portal to dissect the cranial and caudal part of the patent ductus arteriosus. Do not dissect the medial side of the ductus. The surgeon is standing on the dorsal side of the patient. Use large vascular clips to occlude the ductus.

TREATMENT OF PYOTHORAX

Pyothorax represents a challenge for internists and surgeons. Dogs most often present for the treatment of chronic pyothorax. Blood work, auscultation, and basic and advanced imaging technology are not able to differentiate chronic versus acute pyothorax and do not provide reliable information for the optimal treatment in each patient. Dogs are routinely medically managed for 2 to 3 days. If improvements are not obvious after 3 days, surgery is recommended. Dogs seem to respond better to surgical treatment, especially if a mass is present in the lungs or in the mediastinum or if *Actinomyces* is present on cytology.[14]

Thoracoscopy has been recommended in human surgery to assist in the treatment of pyothorax.[15,16] Thoracoscopy is used to explore the entire pleural space, to collect biopsies and cultures, and to debride the mediastinum and every tissue involved in the infectious process.

Approach

Use a transdiaphragmatic approach with the patient in dorsal recumbency to gain access to both sides of the thoracic cavity. Place instrument portals on either side of the thoracic cavity in the eighth or ninth intercostal space close to the sternum.

Surgical Technique

After placement of the portals, the entire mediastinum is dissected from its attachment on the sternum. Use electrocautery or a vessel sealant device for the dissection, as the blood vessels in the mediastinum are usually large and can bleed profusely.

Explore the entire pleural space starting in the thoracic inlet. An angle telescope is recommended because it allows a better visualization of the cranial mediastinum and both sides of each of the lung lobes. Move the telescope caudally to explore each lung lobe. Use a palpation probe and a blunt forceps to manipulate each lung lobe. The patient can be tilted on its left and right side to improve visualization of dorsal part of the right and left hemithoraxes. Also evaluate the pericardium evaluated for involvement in the disease process. It is important to perform an echocardiography before the thoracoscopy to evaluate the status of the pericardium. If the pericardium has increased thickness and if pericardial effusion is present, traditional thoracotomy is more appropriate.

After completing a thorough exploration, the decision can then be taken to pursue with thoracoscopy or to convert to a median sternotomy. If the condition is chronic with multiple adhesions and severe involvement of the pericardium or if lung lobes are involved in the disease process, then a sternotomy is performed. If the condition seems acute with minimal adhesions, biopsies and cultures are taken. Resect as much of the mediastinum as possible under thoracoscopy. Perform pleural lavage under thoracoscopy and place two thoracoscopy tubes under thoracoscopic guidance.

REFERENCES

1. Kovak JR, Ludwig LL, Bergman PJ, et al. Use of thoracoscopy to determine the etiology of pleural effusion in dogs and cats: 18 cases (1998–2001). J Am Vet Med Assoc 2002;221(7):990–4.
2. Borenstein N, Behr L, Chetboul V, et al. Minimally invasive patent ductus arteriosus occlusion in 5 dogs. Vet Surg 2004;33(4):309–13.
3. Brissot HN, Dupre GP, Bouvy BM, et al. Thoracoscopic treatment of bullous emphysema in 3 dogs. Vet Surg 2003;32(6):524–9.
4. Dupre GP, Corlouer JP, Bouvy B. Thoracoscopic pericardectomy performed without pulmonary exclusion in 9 dogs. Vet Surg 2001;30(1):21–7.
5. Jackson J, Richter KP, Launer DP. Thoracoscopic partial pericardiectomy in 13 dogs. J Vet Intern Med 1999;13(6):529–33.
6. Garcia F, Prandi D, Pena T, et al. Examination of the thoracic cavity and lung lobectomy by means of thoracoscopy in dogs. Can Vet J 1998;39(5):285–91.
7. Walsh PJ, Remedios AM, Ferguson JF, et al. Thoracoscopic versus open partial pericardectomy in dogs: comparison of postoperative pain and morbidity. Vet Surg 1999;28(6):472–9.
8. Lansdowne JL, Monnet E, Twedt DC, et al. Thoracoscopic lung lobectomy for treatment of lung tumors in dogs. Vet Surg 2005;34(5):530–5.
9. MacPhail CM, Monnet E, Twedt DC. Thoracoscopic correction of persistent right aortic arch in a dog. J Am Anim Hosp Assoc 2001;37(6):577–81.
10. Radlinsky MG, Mason DE, Biller DS, et al. Thoracoscopic visualization and ligation of the thoracic duct in dogs. Vet Surg 2002;31(2):138–46.
11. Levionnois OL, Bergadano A, Schatzmann U. Accidental entrapment of an endobronchial blocker tip by a surgical stapler during selective ventilation for lung lobectomy in a dog. Vet Surg 2006;35(1):82–5.
12. Kudnig ST, Monnet E, Riquelme M, et al. Effect of positive end-expiratory pressure on oxygen delivery during 1-lung ventilation for thoracoscopy in normal dogs. Vet Surg 2006;35(6):534–42.
13. Enwiller TM, Radlinsky MG, Mason DE, et al. Popliteal and mesenteric lymph node injection with methylene blue for coloration of the thoracic duct in dogs. Vet Surg 2003;32(4):359–64.
14. Rooney MB, Monnet E. Medical and surgical treatment of pyothorax in dogs: 26 cases. J Am Vet Med Assoc 2002;221(1):86–92.
15. Grewal H, Jackson RJ, Wagner CW, et al. Early video-assisted thoracic surgery in the management of empyema. [Review] [30 refs]. Pediatrics 1999;103(5):e63.
16. Roberts JR. Minimally invasive surgery in the treatment of empyema: intraoperative decision making. Ann Thorac Surg 2003;76(1):225–30 [discussion: 229–30].

Complications and Need for Conversion from Thoracoscopy to Thoracotomy in Small Animals

MaryAnn G. Radlinsky, DVM, MS

KEYWORDS
- Thoracoscopy • Complications • Conversion • Thoracotomy

The most common indications for thoracoscopy include mass lesions of the pleura, lungs, lymph nodes, or mediastinum, chronic, undiagnosed pleural effusion, chylothorax, pericardial effusion with or without mass lesions, spontaneous pneumothorax, and persistent right aortic arch (PRAA). Thoracoscopic procedures may be diagnostic or therapeutic. Diagnostic procedures include exploration and biopsy of any of the following: pleura, mediastinum, lymph node, pericardium, lung, and mass lesions of any of the aforementioned structures. Therapeutic procedures include formation of a pericardial window, subtotal pericardectomy, partial, or complete pneumolobectomy, thoracic duct ligation, and ligation and division of the ligamentum arteriosum. The most common complications of thoracoscopy include hemorrhage and trauma to adjacent structures or structures outside the area of visualization within the thoracic cavity. Conversion may be required due to direct complications of thoracoscopy in general, the specific procedure done, anesthetic problems, patient limitations, or prolonged duration of the procedure being done.

GENERAL

Clinicians performing thoracoscopy should be able to perform the same procedures required by the patient by open thoracotomy on an elective or emergent basis. The equipment necessary to perform open thoracotomy should be readily available in the operating suite, and the patient should be adequately prepared and draped for thoracostomy tube placement and thoracotomy. Finocietto retractors, electrocautery, radiosurgery, vascular clip appliers, and sealing devices normally used for open thoracotomy should be in the operating suite ready for immediate use. If the patient is

Department of Small Animal Medicine and Surgery, College of Veterinary Medicine, University of Georgia, 501 DW Brooks Drive, Athens, GA 30602, USA
E-mail address: radlinsk@uga.edu

Vet Clin Small Anim 39 (2009) 977–984
doi:10.1016/j.cvsm.2009.05.006
0195-5616/09/$ – see front matter © 2009 Elsevier Inc. All rights reserved.

placed in dorsal recumbency, an oscillating saw should be in the operating suite for conversion to a median sternotomy. A thoracostomy tube should be placed following every thoracoscopic procedure to monitor for pneumothorax and hemorrhage, which are the most common complications of thoracoscopy.

ANESTHESIA

Mechanical ventilation is a requirement for thoracoscopy. The tidal volume is typically reduced and ventilatory frequency increased during thoracoscopy to provide adequate visualization. Thoracoscopy results in decreased PaO_2, CaO_2, $EtCO_2$, and increased physiologic dead space ventilation, shunt fraction, and $PA-aO_2$.[1] One-lung ventilation results in ipsilateral atelectasis and increases the working space and visual field for thoracoscopy. One-lung ventilation decreased PaO_2 and increased the shunt fraction and $PaCO_2$; positive end expiratory pressure (PEEP) was used in another study to offset the changes that occurred during one-lung ventilation.[2,3] Thoracic insufflation is rarely reported, required, or recommended to further increase working space and visualization during thoracoscopy. Insufflation decreased cardiac output, arterial blood pressure, oxygen saturation, central venous pressure, cardiac output, and heart rate in one study.[4] These experimental studies were performed on healthy animals, and the response to thoracoscopy and the alterations in ventilation needed may not be the same in patients with thoracic or pulmonary disease. Anesthetic complications may necessitate conversion to open thoracotomy to allow adequate ventilation and adequate visualization if larger pulmonary excursions with less atelectasis are needed to maintain proper patient ventilation. Failure to maintain one-lung ventilation may also result in conversion to thoracotomy in a procedure that requires one-lung ventilation.[5] Most thoracoscopic procedures do not require one-lung ventilation, and entrapment of the guide wire associated with an endobronchial blocker is another reported complication of one-lung ventilation used for pneumolobectomy.[6,7] Conversion to thoracotomy was not required in that report.[7]

HEMORRHAGE

Port placement can result in hemorrhage from the intercostal vasculature early in the procedure. The presence of the port in the intercostal space, however, may prevent diagnosis of the problem until the port is removed.[5,8,9] Inspection of the port sites on placement and removal is recommended, as significant hemorrhage from the intercostal vessels can be life threatening if not diagnosed until the animal is recovered from anesthesia.[5] Use of a Veress needle followed by thoracic insufflation does not eliminate the risk of trauma to the lung, heart, vasculature, esophagus, or trachea.[10,11] Damage to the intercostal vessels and nerves can be minimized if ports are placed through a mini-thoracotomy. A skin incision followed by blunt dissection in the center of the intercostal space provides for safe establishment of pneumothorax. Then use a blunt obturater for port placement to further decrease the risk of inadvertent organ trauma. Subsequent ports should be placed in a similar manner, but under endoscopic visualization. Each port site should be evaluated on removal to evaluate for and to decrease postoperative hemorrhage.

Hemorrhage from the intercostal vessels may also occur during pleural biopsy. Ideally, biopsies should be taken where intercostal vessels are not present, which is best done by visualizing the intercostal artery and vein. However, chronicity of pleural effusion and the type of disease process may cause pleural fibrosis, which can obscure the intercostal vessels and nerves. Palpate the ribs with biopsy forceps. Biopsies should be taken from the central region of the chosen intercostal space, making sure to avoid the vasculature and nerves adjacent to the caudal aspect of the ribs, even if they are not visible. Monitor the biopsy sites after collection and take measures to decrease or eliminate hemorrhage as necessary.

Intercostal vessel hemorrhage can be controlled by the same techniques used during open thoracotomy. Apply pressure to the site, and if pressure is insufficient for controlling hemorrhage, electrocautery (mono- or bipolar), vascular clips, suture ligation, or sealing devices may be used. Suction with or without irrigation may also be required for visualization for hemostasis. Failure to eliminate significant intercostal vascular hemorrhage may require conversion to an open approach, during which the vessel(s) should be identified and controlled.

Hemorrhage can also occur from other vessels, depending on the procedure. Vessels associated with the mediastinum, lymph nodes, lung, pericardium, and great vessels (ductus arteriosus), or mass lesions may result in significant hemorrhage. Inflammatory or neoplastic processes may cause increased vascularity within the thorax. Significant dissection and resection of mediastinum and pericardium may be required in the treatment of pyothorax. Mediastinal dissection during thoracoscopy in patients in dorsal recumbency allows the surgeon access to both hemithoraces. Continued hemorrhage from the ventral mediastinum should be controlled to decrease blood loss and to improve visualization by decreasing blood contamination of the endoscope tip. Hemostasis can be achieved thoracoscopically using the methods discussed earlier without converting to thoracotomy, especially as experience is gained with endosurgery.[12] The presence of significant adhesions in cases of chronic pleural effusion or pyothorax may limit visualization because of hemorrhage or interference with the ability to view normal anatomy, causing the surgeon to convert to open thoracotomy.[13]

PNEUMOTHORAX

Pneumothorax maybe the result of inadvertent or visualized lung injury. It is important to manipulate instruments under endoscopic visualization during all parts of the procedure to minimize the risk of pulmonary trauma. A wide view should be maintained, and the port of entry viewed during the introduction of the instruments. The view may be narrowed when the instruments reach the operative target. Establishment of pneumothorax usually provides the atelectasis necessary for most thoracoscopic procedures. If further operative space is necessary, one-lung ventilation on the side of the surgery will cause complete atelectasis of the chosen lung lobes. One-lung ventilation, however, is not commonly required for procedures other than pneumolobectomy.[5,6,13–17] The lungs also respond to altering the position of the body, allowing gravity to displace the lungs away from the operative target. Ports should be placed so that the introduction and removal of instruments during the procedure will result in the lowest risk of pulmonary trauma. During thoracoscopic evaluation of the patient in dorsal recumbency, ports can easily be placed ventral to pulmonary excursions by visualization of the intended port site. Place digital pressure or manipulate a closed instrument at the intended port site before port placement to ensure pulmonary excursions are avoided during the introduction of the instruments. Fan-shaped retractors can be introduced through a port to retract lung tissue during thoracoscopy, which is more commonly required for therapeutic than for diagnostic procedures. Care must be taken to avoid trapping small portions of lung between the blades of the fan-shaped retractor, especially during closure of the device. No instrument should be left unattended or without visualization in the thorax.

Pulmonary trauma can be definitively diagnosed by direct visualization. The thorax can be infused with warm irrigation solution, and the lungs evaluated for air leakage as during open thoracotomy. Damaged areas of lung may be addressed as in open thoracotomy: placement of a thoracostomy tube for small leaks, suturing, Endoloop ligation, staple excision, or complete pneumolobectomy. Conversion to open thoracotomy may or may not be necessary to resolve pulmonary trauma.

INABILITY TO COMPLETE THE INTENDED PROCEDURE

Anesthetic complications, inability to ventilate the patient with the amount of atelectasis required for thoracoscopic visualization, adhesions interfering with visualization, identification of large lesions, unacceptably long duration of a procedure, and inexperience may require the surgeon to convert to an open thoracotomy.[5,13,18] The risk of conversion due to inability to localize or operate on the intended target decreases with an increasing amount of information on procedures and surgeon experience. Most clinicians attend practical educational conferences with laboratory experience before performing thoracoscopic procedures. Starting with exploratory and diagnostic procedures allows familiarization with port placement, instrumentation, and different approaches to the thorax. As experience is gained, therapeutic interventions may be performed. The surgeon can also set a time limit when first performing a new procedure. The procedure may be completed thoracoscopically if adequate operative progress is made during that time period. If adequate progress is not made, conversion to an open thoracotomy may be done, and the surgeon and assistants can assess the difficulties or problems that led to the lack of progress and apply them to subsequent cases. It is wise to avoid overweight animals when first performing thoracoscopic procedures, as mediastinal fat will make anatomic identification more difficult. Entry into the mediastinal fat on placement of a paraxiphoid port will also confuse the surgeon and interferes greatly with visualization, necessitating conversion to thoracotomy. More advanced procedures such as correction of PRAA, patent ductus arteriosus (PDA), and pneumolobectomy have been reported in the veterinary literature with few conversions required, emphasizing the increasing expansion of thoracoscopy and skill of veterinary endoscopists.[5,16,17,19–21]

POSTOPERATIVE PAIN

Thoracoscopy has gained wide acceptance due to the decreased morbidity associated with smaller incisions and lack of rib or sternal retraction.[10] Pressure on the intercostal nerves due to ports used during thoracoscopy may result in some pain after thoracoscopy.[9,21] Local anesthetic placed at each port site should help provide postoperative analgesia. Use of soft, flexible ports may also decrease postoperative pain because they conform to the intercostal space and should apply less pressure on the nerve and adjacent rib during thoracoscopy. Intrapleural application of local anesthetic may also be used to decrease pain and has been deemed safe even after formation of a pericardial window.[22] Increased right ventricular diastolic pressure and systemic vascular resistance occurred in the control and pericardial window groups in that study.[22]

THORACOSCOPIC-ASSISTED PROCEDURES

The use of thoracoscopy may be expanded to assisted procedures to augment the ability of the surgeon to perform more technically challenging procedures and may decrease the need for conversion. The most accepted assisted technique is partial lung lobectomy. After complete inspection of the thorax, including the hilar lymph nodes, the affected portion of lung is exposed by lengthening one port site without rib separation. The lung may then be stapled or sutured for removal. Clip application of PDA has also been reported with an assisted technique with no need for conversion to traditional thoracotomy.[23] The technique has also been used to decrease dissection of the cranio-medial aspect of the ductus to decrease the risk of hemorrhage, but application was limited by ductal size.[21] Complications with these procedures are no different from thoracoscopy or thoracotomy and should be treated similarly.

LITERATURE REVIEW

The veterinary literature reports few cases of conversion from thoracoscopy to thoracotomy. Cases range from simple exploration to invasive techniques.[15,22] In cases of exploration for anatomic evaluation or part of an experimental research protocol, no complications were noted, and thoracoscopy alone did not seem to induce any adhesions.[15,22] When the scope of exploration included biopsies of pleura, pericardium, mass lesions, or pericardium for the diagnosis of persistent pleural effusion, one conversion was required in 18 patients. The conversion was due to the presence of multiple adhesions, which limited thoracoscopic visualization.[13]

More invasive procedures have become the standard of care in veterinary medicine; the most commonly performed thoracoscopic therapeutic technique has been pericardectomy. Complications associated with the procedure were limited to hypercapnia and hypoxemia in one early study that used thoracic insufflation.[10] No conversions to an open approach were required. However, if the pericardectomy allows the heart to herniate through a small window causing cardiac compression or limiting atrial motion, conversion may be required. As surgeons increased their thoracoscopic skills, more refined techniques were developed for pericardectomy.[6] Treatment of PRAA has been described using two different approaches in four dogs, none of which required conversion to thoracotomy.[19,20] In the author's experience, hemorrhage from the transected structure (ie, ductus arteriosus instead of a ligamentum arteriosum) may require conversion to thoracotomy. Experimental ligation of the thoracic duct has also been reported without conversion, despite the need for two-lung ventilation in one dog; normal dogs were placed in sternal recumbency, eliminating pulmonary interference with visualization of the dorsal thorax.[18]

One of the most complex procedures developed is thoracoscopic lung lobectomy. Stapling devices are usually employed, and failure of the device is not solely a thoracoscopic issue. A total of 20 thoracoscopic lung lobectomy cases have been reported, and conversion was required in four dogs with lung tumors.[5,16,17] The conversions were required for intercostal hemorrhage, failure of one-lung ventilation, and poor access to the right middle lung lobe.[5] There were no conversions for cases of spontaneous pneumothorax or experimental lobectomy.[16,17] Improvements in technique and skill may decrease the need for conversions during lobectomy in the future; however, access to the right middle and accessory lung lobes makes excisions difficult.[5]

The human literature describes port site metastasis as another complication of thoracoscopy, which has also been reported in one veterinary case.[24] It is not clear whether port site metastasis is due to persistent exposure of malignant pleural effusion to port sites after surgery or direct transfer of neoplastic cells during withdrawal of specimens, as the use of specimen bags may not completely eliminate port site metastasis.[25] The lack of evidence led some authors to believe that port site metastasis may be related to intrathoracic manipulation of the tumor, rather than direct contact with the site.[26]

Other problems requiring conversion to thoracotomy included unexpected large size of the target lesion, pneumothorax, persistent pleural effusion, and inaccessibility of the lesion.[27] A 1.7% conversion rate was present in 1 study, and complications of thoracoscopy occurred in 17% of patients.[27] Complications were higher in infectious disease states, patients with immunocompromise, and older patients.[27] Complications reported included pleural effusion, self-limiting pneumothorax, and death (0.8%).[27] Conversions were required for chronic fistulae that could not be corrected thoracoscopically or inaccessible lesions.

Other studies of more than 100 people reported complication rates of 0% to 79% depending on the type of procedure.[8,9,12,21,28,29] Reported complications associated with thoracoscopic pulmonary resection, sympathectomy, and splanchnicectomy included anesthesia-related problems, pneumothorax, pleural effusion, ventilatory insufficiency, hemorrhage, empyema, intercostal neuralgia, port site infection, fibrosis, atrial fibrillation, and pulmonary, bronchial, or diaphragmatic trauma.[8,9,12,28,29] Complications of the specific procedures also occurred, but are not included in this discussion. Conversion to thoracotomy occurred 0% to 23% of the time.[8,9,12,28,29] Indications for conversion included equipment problems, anatomic abnormalities, vascular injury, bronchial trauma, identification of more advanced disease than anticipated, inability to identify small pulmonary lesions, pleural adhesions, and the need for further tissue resection.[8,9,12,28,29] One study reported improvement in technique over time and a decrease in the need for conversion as skills were developed.[12]

Thoracoscopy has been reported for PDA ligation, sympathectomy, mediastinal mass excision, diaphragmatic herniorrhaphy, esophagectomy, partial pneumolobectomy, other mass excision in smaller reports of less than 100 people each.[11,30–41] Complication rates ranged from 0% to 22.7% and included trochar site infection, pneumonia, hemothorax, venous thrombosis, cardiac arrhythmias, phrenic nerve damage, and pneumothorax.[11,30–41] Conversions were reported in 0% to 10%, with 6 studies reporting no conversions.[30,32,36,38,40,41] Conversions were required due to hemorrhage associated with sympathectomy, mediastinal mass excision, esophagectomy, and partial pneumolobectomy.[30,31,36,38,40,41] Decreased oxygen saturation resulted in conversion to thoracotomy in a patient undergoing diaphragmatic herniorrhaphy.[34] Lesions being too deep in the pulmonary parenchyma led to conversion in 4% of patients in one study that evaluated excision of small (<3 cm) pulmonary nodules.[39] Other reasons for conversion included organ perforation, Veress needle trauma, hemorrhage, difficulty in anatomic identification, and hypercapnia in one study that evaluated thoracoscopy and laparoscopy in pediatric patients.[11]

SUMMARY

The equipment and skill required for conversion should be considered before undertaking any thoracoscopic procedure. Complications and the need for conversion to thoracotomy in veterinary patients undergoing thoracoscopic procedures are usually related to anesthesia, impaired visualization due to hemorrhage or pleural adhesions, significant hemorrhage, and pulmonary trauma. As experience is gained, complications and the need for conversion to thoracotomy may decrease, as complications may be dealt with thoracoscopically. Further reports in the veterinary literature will elucidate the importance of patient selection and procedures done and how each relates to potential complications and the need for conversion.

REFERENCES

1. Kudnig ST, Monnet E, Riquelme M, et al. Cardiopulmonary effects of thoracoscopy in anesthetized normal dogs. Vet Anaesth Analg 2004;31:121–8.

2. Kudnig ST, Monnet E, Riquelme M, et al. Effect of one-lung ventilation on oxygen delivery in anesthetized dogs with an open thoracic cavity. Am J Vet Res 2003;64: 443–8.

3. Kudnig ST, Monnet E, Riquelme M, et al. Effect of end-expiratory pressure on oxygen delivery during 1-lung ventilation for thoracoscopy in normal dogs. Vet Surg 2006;35(6):534–42.

4. Daly CM, Swalec-Tobias K, Tobias AH, et al. Cardiopulmonary effects of intrathoracic insufflation in dogs. J Am Anim Hosp Assoc 2002;28:515–20.

5. Lansdowne JL, Monnet E, Twedt DC, et al. Thoracoscopic lung lobectomy for treatment of lung tumors in dogs. Vet Surg 2005;34:530–5.

6. Dupre GP, Corlouer JP, Bouvy B. Thoracoscopic pericardectomy performed without pulmonary exclusion in 9 dogs. Vet Surg 2001;30:21–7.

7. Levionnois OL, Bergadano A, Schatzmann U. Accidental entrapment of an endobronchial blocker tip by a surgical stapler during selective ventilation for lung lobectomy in a dog. Vet Surg 2006;35:82–5.

8. Baghdadi S, Abbas MH, Albouz F, et al. Systematic review of the role of thoracoscopic splanchnicectomy in palliating the pain of patients with chronic pancreatitis. Surg Endosc 2008;22:580–8.

9. Solaini L, Prusciano F, Bagioni P, et al. Video-assisted thoracic surgery (VATS) of the lung. Analysis of intraoperative and postoperative complications over 15 years and review of the literature. Surg Endosc 2008;22:298–310.

10. Walsh PJ, Remedios AM, Ferguson JF, et al. Thoracoscopic versus open partial pericardectomy in dogs; comparison of postoperative pain and morbidity. Vet Surg 1999;28:472–9.

11. Esposito C, Mattioli G, Monguzzi GL, et al. Complications and conversions of pediatric videosurgery. Surg Endosc 2002;16:795–8.

12. Congregado M, Merchan RJ, Gallardo G, et al. Video-assisted thoracic surgery (VATS) lobectomy: 13 years' experience. Surg Endosc 2008;22: 1852–7.

13. Kovak JR, Ludwig LL, Bergman PJ, et al. Use of thoracoscopy to determine the etiology of pleural effusion in dogs and cats: 18 cases (1998–2001). J Am Vet Med Assoc 2002;221:990–4.

14. DeRycke LM, Gielen IM, Polis I, et al. Thoracoscopic anatomy of dogs positioned in lateral recumbency. J Am Anim Hosp Assoc 2001;37:543–8.

15. Jerram RM, Fossum TW, Berridge BR, et al. The efficacy of mechanical abrasion and talc slurry as methods of pluerodesis in normal dogs. Vet Surg 1999;28: 322–32.

16. Garcia F, Prandi D, Pena T, et al. Examination of the thoracic cavity and lung lobectomy by means of thoracoscopy in dogs. Can Vet J 1998;39:285–91.

17. Brissot HN, Dupre GP, Bouvy BM, et al. Thoracoscopic treatment of bullous emphysema in 3 dogs. Vet Surg 2003;32:524–9.

18. Radlinsky MG, Mason DE, Biller DS, et al. Thoracoscopic visualization and ligation of the thoracic duct in dogs. Vet Surg 2002;31:128–46.

19. MacPhail CM, Monnet E, Twedt DC. Thoracoscopic correction of persistent right aortic arch in a dog. J Am Anim Hosp Assoc 2001;37:577–81.

20. Isakow K, Fowler D, Walsh P. Video-assisted thoracoscopic division of the ligamentum arteriosum in two dogs with persistent right aortic arch. J Am Vet Med Assoc 2000;217:1333–6.

21. Sciuchetti J, Corti F, Ballabio D, et al. Results, side effects and complications after thoracoscopic sympathetic block by clamping. The Monza clinical experience. Clin Auton Res 2008;18:80–3.

22. Bernard F, Kudnig ST, Monnet E. Hemodynamic effects of interpleural lidocaine and bupivacaion combination in anesthetized dogs with and without an open pericardium. Vet Surg 2006;35:252–8.
23. Borenstein N, Behr L, Chetboul V, et al. Minimally invasive patent ductus arteriosus occlusion in 5 dogs. Vet Surg 2004;33:309–13.
24. Brisson BA, Reggit F, Bienzle D. Portal site metastasis of invasive mesothelioma after diagnostic thoracoscopy in a dog. J Am Vet Med Assoc 2006;229(6):980–3.
25. Parekh K, Rusch V, Bains M, et al. VATS port site recurrence: a technique dependent problem. Ann Surg Oncol 2001;8:175–8.
26. Rieger R, Schrenk P, Wayand W. Thoracoscopic resection of a malignant pulmonary lesion – the use of a specimen bag may not prevent tumor seeding to the chest wall. Acta Chir Austriaca 1997;29:55–7.
27. Winter H, Meimarakis G, Pirker M, et al. Predictors of general complications after video-assisted thoracoscopic surgical procedures. Surg Endosc 2008;22:640–5.
28. Roviaro G, Varoli F, Vergani C, et al. Video-assisted thoracoscopic major pulmonary resections. Surg Endosc 2004;18:1551–8.
29. Ambrogi MC, Dini P, Boni G, et al. A strategy for thoracoscopic resection of small pulmonary nodules. Surg Endosc 2005;19:1644–7.
30. Dutta S, Mihailovic A, Benson L, et al. Thoracoscopic ligation versus coil occlusion for patent ductus arteriosus: a matched cohort study of outcomes and cost. Surg Endosc 2008;22:1643–8.
31. Lee AD, Agarwal S, Sadhu D. A 7-year experience with thoracoscopic sympathectomy for critical upper limb ischemia. World J Surg 2006;30:1644–7.
32. Miyaji K, Ka K, Okamoto H, et al. One-lung ventilation for video-assisted thoracoscopic interruption of patent ductus arteriosus. Surg Today 2004;24:1006–9.
33. Dmitriev EG, Sigal EI. Thoracoscopic surgery in the management of mediastinal masses. Surg Endosc 1996;10:718–20.
34. Shalaby R, Gabr K, Al-Saied G, et al. Thoracoscopic repair of diaphragmatic hernia in neonates and children: a new simplified technique. Pediatr Surg Int 2008;24:543–7.
35. Gossot D, Cattan P, Fritsch S, et al. Can the morbidity of esophagectomy be reduced by the thoracoscopic approach? Surg Endosc 1995;9:1113–5.
36. Yim APC. Video-assisted thoracoscopic suturing of apical bullae; an alternative to staple resection in the management of primary spontaneous pneumothorax. Surg Endosc 1995;9:1013–6.
37. Shiono H, Inoue A, Tomiyama N, et al. Safer video-assisted thoracoscopic thymectomy after location of thymic veins with multidetector computed tomography. Surg Endosc 2006;20:1419–22.
38. Esposito C, Lima M, Mattioli G, et al. Thoracoscopic surgery in the management of pediatric malignancies: a multicentric survey of the Italian Society of Videosurgery in Infancy. Surg Endosc 2007;21:1772–5.
39. Pittet O, Christodoulou C, Pezzetta E, et al. Video-assisted thoracoscopic resection of small pulmonary nodule after computed tomography-guided localization with a hook-wire system. World J Surg 2007;31:575–8.
40. Bachmann K, Burkhardt D, Schreiter I, et al. Long-term outcome and quality of life after open and thoracoscopic thymectomy for myasthenia gravis: analysis of 131 patients. Surg Endosc 2008;22:2470–7.
41. Cohen Z, Shinhar D, Kurzbart E, et al. Laproscopic and thoracoscopic surgery in children and adolescents: a 3-year experience. Pediatr Surg Int 1997;12:356–9.

Index

Note: Page numbers of article titles are in **boldface** type.

A

Adrenalectomy, laparoscopic, in dogs and cats, 935–939
Airway(s), evaluation of, in dogs and cats, procedures for, **869–880**
Anesthesia/anesthetics
    for endoscopy in small animals, **839–848**
        colonoscopy, 843–844
        general considerations, 839–840
        laparoscopy, 844–845
        laryngoscopy/tracheoscopy, 840–842
        rhinoscopy, 844
        thoracoscopy, 846–847
        upper gastrointestinal endoscopy, 842–843
    for exploratory thoracoscopy in small animals, 957–958
    for thoracoscopy in small animals, complications of, 980
    for tracheobronchoscopy in dogs and cats, 872–873

B

BAL. See *Bronchoalveolar lavage (BAL)*.
Biopsy(ies)
    excisional, in laparoscopic organ biopsy, in small animals, 916
    in airway evaluation, in dogs and cats, 876
    intestinal, laparoscopy in, in small animals, 909–910
    laparoscopic, in small animals, 912–917
    needle, in laparoscopic organ biopsy, in small animals, 913–916
Biopsy cup forceps, in laparoscopic organ biopsy, in small animals, 912
Bronchial brushing, in airway evaluation in dogs and cats, 876
    cytology of, 878
Bronchoalveolar lavage (BAL), in airway evaluation in dogs and cats, 875–876
    cytology of, 877–878

C

Camera, in endoscopy, 823
Cat(s)
    advanced laparoscopic procedures in, **927–941**. See also *Laparoscopy, advanced procedures, in dogs and cats.*
    airway evaluation in
        BAL in, 875–878
        biopsy in, 876
        bronchial brushing in, 876, 878

Vet Clin Small Anim 39 (2009) 985–991
doi:10.1016/S0195-5616(09)00109-0
0195-5616/09/$ – see front matter © 2009 Elsevier Inc. All rights reserved.

ur issues help you manage *yours.*

very year brings you new clinical challenges.

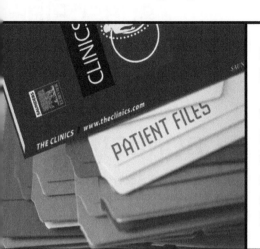

Every **Clinics** issue brings you **today's best thinking** on the challenges you face.

Whether you purchase these issues individually, or order an annual subscription (which includes searchable access to past issues online), the **Clinics** offer you an efficient way to update your know how…one issue at a time.

DISCOVER THE CLINICS IN YOUR SPECIALTY!

Veterinary Clinics of North America: Equine Practice.
Publishes three times a year.
ISSN 0749-0739.

Veterinary Clinics of North America: Exotic Animal Practice.
Publishes three times a year.
ISSN 1094-9194.

Veterinary Clinics of North America: Food Animal Practice.
Publishes three times a year.
ISSN 0749-0720.

Veterinary Clinics of North America: Small Animal Practice.
Publishes bimonthly.
ISSN 0195-5616.

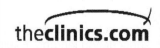

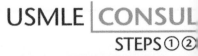

Moving?

Make sure your subscription moves with you!

To notify us of your new address, find your **Clinics Account Number** (located on your mailing label above your name), and contact customer service at:

Email: journalscustomerservice-usa@elsevier.com

800-654-2452 (subscribers in the U.S. & Canada)
314-447-8871 (subscribers outside of the U.S. & Canada)

Fax number: 314-447-8029

Elsevier Health Sciences Division
Subscription Customer Service
3251 Riverport Lane
Maryland Heights, MO 63043

*To ensure uninterrupted delivery of your subscription, please notify us at least 4 weeks in advance of move.

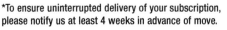

Printed and bound by CPI Group (UK) Ltd, Croydon, CR0 4YY

03/10/2024

01040444-0012